Dementia

A Global Approach

Dementia

A Global Approach

Edited by

Ennapadam S. Krishnamoorthy
The Institute of Neurological Sciences, VHS Hospital, Chennai, India

Martin J. Prince
Institute of Psychiatry, London, UK

Jeffrey L. Cummings
Neurological Institute of Cleveland Clinic Foundation, Las Vegas, USA

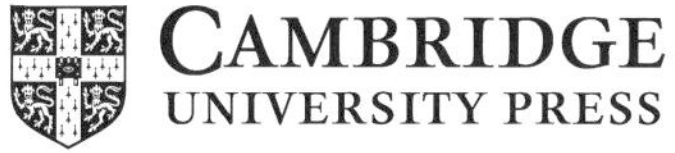

CAMBRIDGE UNIVERSITY PRESS
Cambridge, New York, Melbourne, Madrid, Cape Town, Singapore,
São Paulo, Delhi, Dubai, Tokyo, Mexico City

Cambridge University Press
The Edinburgh Building, Cambridge CB2 8RU, UK

Published in the United States of America by Cambridge University Press, New York

www.cambridge.org
Information on this title: www.cambridge.org/9780521857765

First published 2010

Printed in the United Kingdom at the University Press, Cambridge

A catalog record for this publication is available from the British Library

Library of Congress Cataloging in Publication data
Dementia: a global approach / edited by Ennapadam S. Krishnamoorthy, Martin J. Prince, Jeffrey L. Cummings.
p. cm.
Includes bibliographical references and index.
ISBN 978-0-521-85776-5 (hardback)
1. Dementia. I. Krishnamoorthy, Ennapadam S., 1966– II. Prince, Martin (Martin James), 1960–
III. Cummings, Jeffrey L., 1948–
[DNLM: 1. Dementia – epidemiology. 2. Cross-Cultural Comparison. 3. Dementia – therapy.
WM 220 D376313 2010]
RC521.D4527 2010
616.8′3–dc22 2010006226

ISBN 978-0-521-85776-5 Hardback

Contents

Contributors

Suvarna Alladi
Department of Neurology, Nizam's Institute of Medical Sciences, Hyderabad, India

Thaddeus Alfonso
The Institute of Neurological Sciences, VHS Hospital, Chennai, India

David Ames
National Ageing Research Institute, Parkville and Academic Unit for Psychiatry of Old Age, University of Melbourne Department of Psychiatry, St George's Hospital, Kew, Victoria, Australia

J. V. Bowler
Department of Neurology, Royal Free Hospital, London, UK

Helen Chiu
Department of Psychiatry, The Chinese University of Hong Kong, Hong Kong Special Administrative Region, China

Jeffrey L. Cummings
Cleveland Clinic Lou Ruvo Center for Neurotherapeutics and Translational Research, Lou Ruvo Center for Brain Health, Neurological Institute of Cleveland Clinic Foundation, Las Vegas, NV, USA

Alan D. Dangour
Nutrition and Public Health Intervention Research Unit, Department of Epidemiology and Population Health, London School of Hygiene & Tropical Medicine, London, UK

Annabel Dodds
Institute of Neurology, University College London, London, UK

Eleanor Flynn
Medical Education Unit, Faculty of Medicine, University of Melbourne, Parkville, Victoria, Australia

Keith Gomez
The Institute of Neurological Sciences, VHS Hospital, Chennai, India

Mariella Guerra
Institute of Psychiatry, De Crespigny Park, London, UK

Kathleen S. Hall
Department of Psychiatry, Indiana University School of Medicine, Indianapolis, IN, USA

Hugh Hendrie
Department of Psychiatry, Indiana School of Medicine, Indianapolis, IN, USA

Kua Ee Heok
Department of Psychological Medicine, National University of Singapore, Singapore

Akira Homma
Center for Dementia Care Research in Tokyo, Tokyo, Japan

Vijayan Joy
National Institute of Mental Health and Neurosciences (NIMHANS), Bangalore, India

S. Kalyanasundaram
The Richmond Fellowship Society, Bangalore, India

Ennapadam S. Krishnamoorthy
The Institute of Neurological Sciences, VHS Hospital, Chennai, India

Julia Lane
Bloomfield Hospital, Orange, Australia

Demetris Pillas
Imperial College London and ESRC International Centre for Life Course Studies in Society and Health, London, UK

Martin J. Prince
Institute of Psychiatry, De Crespigny Park, London, UK

Sadanand Rajkumar
Rural Clinical School, University of Sydney, Orange, Australia

Seethalakshmi Ramanathan
Department of Psychiatry, KEM Hospital, Mumbai, India

Jacob Roy Kuriakose
Alzheimer's Related Disorders Society of India, Kunnankulam, Kerala, India

P. Satishchandra
National Institute of Mental Health and Neurosciences (NIMHANS), Bangalore, India

Caroline Selai
University College London – Institute of Neurology, National Hospital for Neurology and Neurosurgery, London, UK

Vorapun Senanarong
Division of Neurology, Department of Medicine, Faculty of Medicine Siriraj Hospital, Mahidol University, Bangkok, Thailand

R. Stewart
King's College London (Institute of Psychiatry), De Crespigny Park, London, UK

Joshua Tsoh
Department of Psychiatry, The Chinese University of Hong Kong, Hong Kong Special Administrative Region, China

Ricardo Uauy
Nutrition and Public Health Intervention Research Unit, Department of Epidemiology and Population Health, London School of Hygiene & Tropical Medicine, London, UK

Richard Uwakwe
Faculty of Medicine, Nnamdi Azikiwe University, Nigeria

Marc Wortmann
Alzheimer's Disease International, London, UK

Xin Yu
Institute of Mental Health, Peking University, Beijing, China

The aging brain and mind: cultural and anthropological perspectives

Kua Ee Heok

Introduction

Population aging in the twenty-first century is the preeminent demographic phenomenon in Asia. In countries like Japan and Singapore, low fertility rate and better health care are factors explaining the graying of the population. Demographic aging is however becoming a pan-Asian phenomenon with fertility rates falling and health care improving across the globe including the most populous nations, China and India.

The perception of old age differs in different societies and cultures. Nonetheless, it is influenced to a large extent by retirement legislation. When people retired at 55 years, those who were 56 years of age were considered old. Today with the retirement ages ranging from 60 to 65, the 56-year-olds are no longer considered senior citizens.

In population statistics, elderly people are often classified as a single demographic group; but even within the same country or community they are not homogenous. Besides differences in health and social needs, there is also the cultural divide. Policy makers are aware that in a few years, the majority of "baby-boomers" will reach retirement age – they will be the "new-old." In Asia, there are apparent differences between the present elderly population and the "new-old" in perception of old age – the former are more steeped in tradition and culture and the latter less influenced by traditional values. Compared to their aged parents, the "new-old" are better educated and have grown up in an era of economic progress.

Cultural beliefs and aging

Aspirations of old age in the Asian community are influenced by cultural beliefs. For more than a thousand years, Chinese families have worshipped in their homes three deities who personify longevity, happiness, and wealth. They represent their aspirations – to live to a

Dementia: A Global Approach, ed. Ennapadam S. Krishnamoorthy, Martin J. Prince, and Jeffrey L. Cummings. Published by Cambridge University Press.

ripe old age, have sufficient finances, and enjoy good health. Many communities around the world also harbor similar aspirations. Embedded in the Asian tradition of filial piety is the expectation that children should take care of their aged parents and provide financial, social, and emotional support. Such tradition is still present in many agrarian communities but with the rapid global economic changes and the movement of the young working population from rural to urban industrialized communities, and across national boundaries, the care of the elderly is becoming a problem that is rapidly achieving critical proportions. In the cities, the fragmentation of the extended family has an impact on the elderly at home.

In many cultures, the notions of health and old age are entrenched in customs and religious beliefs. Since ancient times, spirituality and health are closely associated. The art of healing and the role of the priest are linked. In Asian countries, with advances in modern medicine, the doctor has a lead role in health care; however, among the elderly, traditional healers and priests are still consulted first [1]. In traditional Chinese medicine, the therapeutic alliance between the patient and the healer hinges on the shared cultural belief of "yin–yang," a bipolarity that is opposite and complementary. When this homeostasis is disrupted, illness may result, and a prescription of herbs is necessary to restore the balance of the "yin" and "yang." In a community study of illness behavior in Singapore, it was found that about 25.3% of elderly people took traditional medicine to prevent ill health and during illness [2].

For many centuries, Chinese and Koreans have believed there is an association between longevity and the consumption of ginkgo biloba. In some Chinese cuisines, the ginkgo nut is an essential ingredient in the recipe not just for the taste or flavor but also its medicinal value. In recent years, ginkgo biloba extract has been sold in traditional medicine shops and pharmacies to prevent memory impairment. There are many other varieties of herbs, which are often brewed and consumed as health supplements by elderly people.

In Chinese culture, exercise is emphasized as a method to restore the "yin–yang" equilibrium in old age. "Tai-chi" is a popular martial art exercise among elderly people in many Asian countries – it is a lifestyle habit for preservation and restoration of physical and mental health. Such practice is also observed in other countries like India, Japan, and Korea, where elderly people are often seen in parks or gardens, performing the graceful exercises.

Life satisfaction

Life satisfaction is a subjective perception of one's overall assessment of life quality and general well-being from comparing one's aspiration to actual life achievement and condition. It implies a perspective of past, present, and future life condition. The major determinants of life satisfaction include education, occupation, marital status, health, income, support from primary groups (family and friends), and participation in social and leisure activities. Life satisfaction is multifactorial and varies with individuals. There are also differences between gender, age groups, social class, and ethnicity.

In a survey in 2004 of elderly Chinese in Singapore [3], factors associated with life satisfaction were explored including reasons for satisfaction. Of the 2325 respondents, 1646 (70.8%) expressed overall satisfaction as being "excellent or good" and 679 (29.2%) as " fair or poor." Elderly individuals with "excellent or good" life satisfaction were married; lived with their families; and were more likely to exercise, read the daily papers, attend the church or temple regularly, look after their grandchildren, and visit community centers or clubs. About 42% stated the main reason for satisfaction was physical comfort, e.g., owning a house, television, refrigerator, radio, washing machine, etc. The second and third reasons were good health and family relationships.

Another study of elderly Chinese conducted ten years earlier [4] showed that 72% felt satisfied and in this group the main reasons were good family relationship (41%), physical comfort (29%), and good health (23%). There is thus an important change in the ranking of life satisfaction after a mere ten-year period. In the 1994 study, the participating elderly were mainly immigrants with low income and dependent on their families to take care of them. In the 2004 study, the participating elderly were second-generation Chinese who were more financially secure and lived in better homes.

The association between spirituality and life satisfaction is observed in the Asian elderly, who regularly visit the temple, mosque, or church. The connection between spirituality and health is complex. It could be that those who attend religious services experience lower levels of anxiety or depression and they also benefit from the social support systems that religious places, churches, temples, and mosques offer. In general most religious beliefs tend to disapprove risky behavior like excessive drinking or smoking, and religious teachings may improve people's ability to cope with stress in late life.

Mood and cognitive decline

A review of the prevalence of depression in late life [5] indicated that the rates were higher for European and American than Asian countries. A possible explanation of the lower prevalence in Singapore and Japan is the sociocultural influence on the perception of elderly people. The emphasis on respect for the elderly and family support may be crucial in elevating the status of old people and minimizing stress in old age. It is undeniable that care and respect of elderly people are values common in most communities, but the practice and expression of such values may vary with ethnicity.

In the Singapore study [6], many of the elderly tended to congregate daily along the common corridors of their flats. They were bonded by clanship ties and a common worry of the depressed Chinese elderly concerning family relationships.

Cultural perception of illness, societal attitude towards the elderly, and family support may explain health-seeking behavior. Most of the elderly in Singapore live in high-rise public housing estates and they prefer to consult traditional healers, who are popular with the elderly not only because of the accessibility of their service but also because they share the same sociocultural beliefs about illness and health. The constellation of symptoms is explained to the patient as due to an excess of "ying" or "yang." A powerful therapeutic factor is the rapport between the patient and the healer, who is able to explain the symptoms using the sociocultural belief system the patient is familiar with. To the elderly Chinese, depressive symptoms like poor appetite, lethargy, or poor sleep are interpreted as due to a "weakness of mental energy." The traditional healer understands the ethos of the subculture and consulting one also avoids the stigma of being labeled a "mental patient," as would happen when they see the doctor in the psychiatric clinic [7].

In the Japanese or Chinese vocabulary, the term "dementia" implies "stupidity" or "mindlessness" – it is humiliating to elderly people. Consequently, many elderly people are reluctant to seek medical consultation because of the stigma. Recently there have been attempts by the Japanese and Chinese medical communities to agree on a more appropriate word.

Assessment of memory impairment in late life at the primary care clinic has been difficult because of limitations in the assessment instruments available. Many existing clinical memory tests lack adequate normative data, reliability, and validity. A brief questionnaire is needed to screen for cognitive change among elderly people in the community, clinic, and hospital. Currently, there are a few of these instruments, including the Mini-Mental State Examination or MMSE [8] and Kahn's Short Portable Mental Status Questionnaire or MSQ [9]. The validity of these tests is doubtful in a different cultural setting where literacy is low.

We have constructed a screening questionnaire called the Elderly Cognitive Assessment Questionnaire or ECAQ [10] for the detection of dementia by the primary care doctor or nurse. The ECAQ assesses two aspects of cognitive function, memory and orientation/information, and has a maximum score of 10 points. The questionnaire can be completed in 10 minutes and is not significantly biased towards educational attainment. The ECAQ is now used by many primary care doctors in Singapore, Malaysia, and Indonesia.

Caring for the frail elderly

There is a growing concern about caring for an increasing number of frail elderly in Asia. This concern is not only because of an increasing number of the elderly but also a diminishing number of carers. Traditionally, carers are the women in the family. The present dilemma emanates partly because of the social transformation in the Asian family. Young couples in the cities prefer to live away from their parents because of the constraint of space in high-rise apartments. Women are better educated now and prefer to go out to work rather than to remain at home. Another factor contributing to the diminishing number of carers is the decrease in the family size – most families today have only one or two children.

Caring for dementia patients is taxing – physically and mentally. A study in Singapore showed that about 56% of family caregivers had symptoms of anxiety and depression related to the stress of caring [11].

Many carers have to work fewer hours, take unpaid leave, or stop working altogether. Family members who have positive feelings towards the patient will be more willing to accept their caregiving role. In Asian countries, the caregivers rely more on family support than on formal geriatric services. Although there are only a few old people's homes or day centers, families may not be eager to use these services because to send an elderly relative to these centers implies a failure of responsibility.

However, with the change in the family structure, many carers may have to turn to the community services.

Policy makers are increasingly aware of the fact that family caregiving is not cost-free. Most retirees do not have pensions and are financially dependent on their children. Caring for the frail elderly in Asia will in all likelihood continue to rest with the family for many years to come. Caregivers may need to seek help outside the home. Support networks typically have the family as the core but should also include friends, neighbours, and home help. Community and governmental support is necessary to alleviate the burden of the family.

Future challenges

The exponential increase in the number of elderly people – the "new-old" – will pose tremendous challenges to health and social services in the near future. In developing and developed countries, the economic impact is sometimes viewed with gloom. This cohort of elderly are better educated than the previous generation and capable of making a strong contribution to society years beyond their official retirement. They should therefore be viewed as a valuable resource – an asset that can benefit the larger community. Their skills and talents should be recognized for gainful employment or voluntarism. The retirement age could increase beyond 65 years if their health permits. Because life expectancy has increased, the majority of the "new-old" workers will not be retiring as early as expected – if there is no pension scheme, it is doubtful whether they have enough money after retirement to enjoy the autumn years. Working in retirement, an oxymoron, may in fact be a reality.

Because of the changes taking place in family structure, more Asian elderly may be living alone in future and cannot expect much support from close relatives. Caring for the elderly with dementia at home will therefore pose many problems. Some of the issues affecting the quality of life of the dementia patient have been identified in a recent Asian seminar; these include inadequate human and financial resources, lack of training for formal caregivers, and lack of support for informal carers [12]. While the Chinese elderly may well continue to worship the three deities for longevity, happiness, and health, it is only the former that they may be assured of, in the years to come.

References

1. Kua EH, Tan CH. Traditional Chinese medicine in psychiatric practice in Singapore. *Int Psychiatry* 2005; **8**: 7–9.
2. Ng TP, Tan CH, Kua EH. The use of Chinese herbal medicines and their correlates in Chinese older adults: the Singapore Chinese Longitudinal Aging Study. *Age Ageing* 2004; **33**: 135–42.
3. Kua EH, Ng TP, Goh LG. *Long Lives*. Singapore, Armour Publishing, 2004.
4. Kua EH. *Ageing and Old Age*. Singapore, Singapore University Press, 1994.
5. Beekman ATF, Copeland JRM, Prince MJ. Review of community prevalence of depression in later life. *Br J Psychiatry* 1999; **174**: 304–6.
6. Kua EH. A community study of mental disorders in elderly Singaporean Chinese using the GMS-AGECAT package. *Aust N Z J Psychiatry* 1992; **26**: 502–6.

7. Kua EH. The depressive elderly Chinese living in the community: a five-year follow-up study. *Int J Geriatr Psychiatry* 1993; **8**: 427–30.
8. Folstein MF, Folstein SE, McHugh PR. Mini-Mental State. A practical method of grading the cognitive state of patients for the clinician. *J Psychiatr Res* 1975; **12**: 189–98.
9. Kahn RL, Goldfarb AL, Pollark M, Peck A. Brief objective measures for the determination of mental status in the aged. *Am J Psychiatry* 1960; **117**: 326–9.
10. Kua EH, Ko SM. A questionnaire to screen for cognitive impairment among elderly people in developing countries. *Acta Psychiatr Scand* 1992; **85**: 119–22.
11. Kua EH, Tan SL. Stress of caregivers of dementia patients in the Singapore Chinese family. *Int J Geriatr Psychiatry* 1997; **12**: 466–9.
12. Chiu E, Chiu H. Dementia in Asia. *Int Psychogeriatr* 2005; **17**: 1–2.

Mild cognitive impairment: current concepts and cross-cultural issues

Seethalakshmi Ramanathan and
Ennapadam S. Krishnamoorthy

Introduction

Increasing longevity has heightened the need to understand the cure and importantly, prevention of disorders linked to aging. The concept of cognitive impairment can be traced back to 2200 BC in the writings of Ptahhotep. Kral [1,2] in 1958 drew attention to the clinical significance of age-related changes in memory. He differentiated between the benign nature of senescent forgetfulness (BSF) and the "amnestic syndrome." Since then numerous definitions have been developed to describe cognitive changes associated with aging. A National Institute of Mental Health work group [3] proposed the concept of age-associated memory impairment (AAMI); these criteria were subsequently revised [4] leading to the concepts of age-consistent memory impairment (ACMI) and late-life forgetfulness (LLF). In 1994, an International Psychogeriatric Association (IPA) task force in collaboration with the World Health Organization (WHO) proposed the concept of age-associated cognitive decline (AACD) [5]. This identifies persons with subjectively and objectively evidenced cognitive decline that is not impairing enough to warrant the diagnosis of dementia and specifies the cognitive domains of memory and learning, attention, and concentration; thinking, language, and visuospatial functioning. Cognitive impairment no dementia (CIND) [6] was defined as a state characterized by lower cognitive performance than would be expected given the age and educational attainment of the person.

The modern concept of "MCI"

Mild cognitive impairment (MCI) primarily identifies an individual with a deteriorating cognitive functioning that is not severe enough to warrant the diagnosis of dementia. It has

Dementia: A Global Approach, ed. Ennapadam S. Krishnamoorthy, Martin J. Prince, and Jeffrey L. Cummings.
Published by Cambridge University Press.

been defined as a Clinical Dementia Rating (Scale) (CDR) stage of 0.5 [7] or Global Deterioration Score (GDS) of 3 [8]. The CDR 0.5 is also compatible with a diagnosis of mild dementia and has largely been criticized for being too inclusive. Proponents for CDR argue that in subjects with MCI, most of the decline is accounted for by memory deficits with minimal functional deficits; their mean CDR sum of boxes is 1.5. Against this, patients with very mild Alzheimer's disease (AD) have a mean CDR sum of boxes score of 3.3, indicating impairment in functional domains as well. This however fails to take into account the considerable heterogeneity in the presentation of MCI. The GDS 3 on the other hand states "subtle cognitive impairment in executive functioning that affects complex occupational and social activities," thereby including other cognitive elements too. However, both GDS and CDR remain severity scales rather than clinically useful definitions [8]. Petersen and colleagues further operationalized these criteria [9]

1. Memory complaint
2. Normal activities of daily living
3. Normal general cognitive function
4. Abnormal memory for age
5. Undemented

However, all the above criteria account for clinical and informant information. A third neuropsychological dimension was added by the European Consortium Task-force in the "MCI Syndrome" [10]

1. Cognitive complaint emanating from the patient and/or his/her family,
2. The subject and/or informant report of a decline in cognitive functioning relative to previous abilities during the past year,
3. Cognitive disorders evidenced by clinical evaluation: impairment in memory and/or another cognitive domain,
4. Cognitive impairment does not have major repercussions on daily life. However, the subject may report difficulties concerning complex day-to-day activities,
5. No dementia.

The European Consortium and other researchers [11] have also identified MCI as a heterogeneous condition with varied presentations, etiologies, and prognoses and have recognized the need to further subclassify MCI on clinical and etiopathogenic grounds.

The clinical classification of MCI:

1. Amnestic (a-MCI) [12]
   Memory complaint usually corroborated by an informant
   Objective memory impairment for age
   Essentially preserved general cognitive function
   Largely intact functional activities
   Not demented
2. Multiple domain (md-MCI)
   Amnestic
   Non-amnestic
3. Single non-amnestic domain.

The etiopathogenic classification of MCI:

1. Neurodegenerative disease – pre-Alzheimer's disease MCI, Lewy body dementia, frontotemporal dementia, and focal atrophy

2. Cognitive disorders corresponding to vascular lesions – vascular pre-dementia MCI. (Vascular MCI/CIND has been identified as mild cognitive disorders that occur after stroke and may progress to more severe cognitive dysfunction.)
3. Mixed dementia
4. Dysphoric or dysthymic disorders – anxiety or depressive syndrome.

A simple algorithm for a complete diagnosis of MCI has been proposed as in Figure 2.1 [12,13].

Epidemiology of MCI

Memory complaints are a common feature among the elderly, with prevalence rates ranging from 25% to over 50%. Prevalence rates of MCI vary depending on the criteria used for

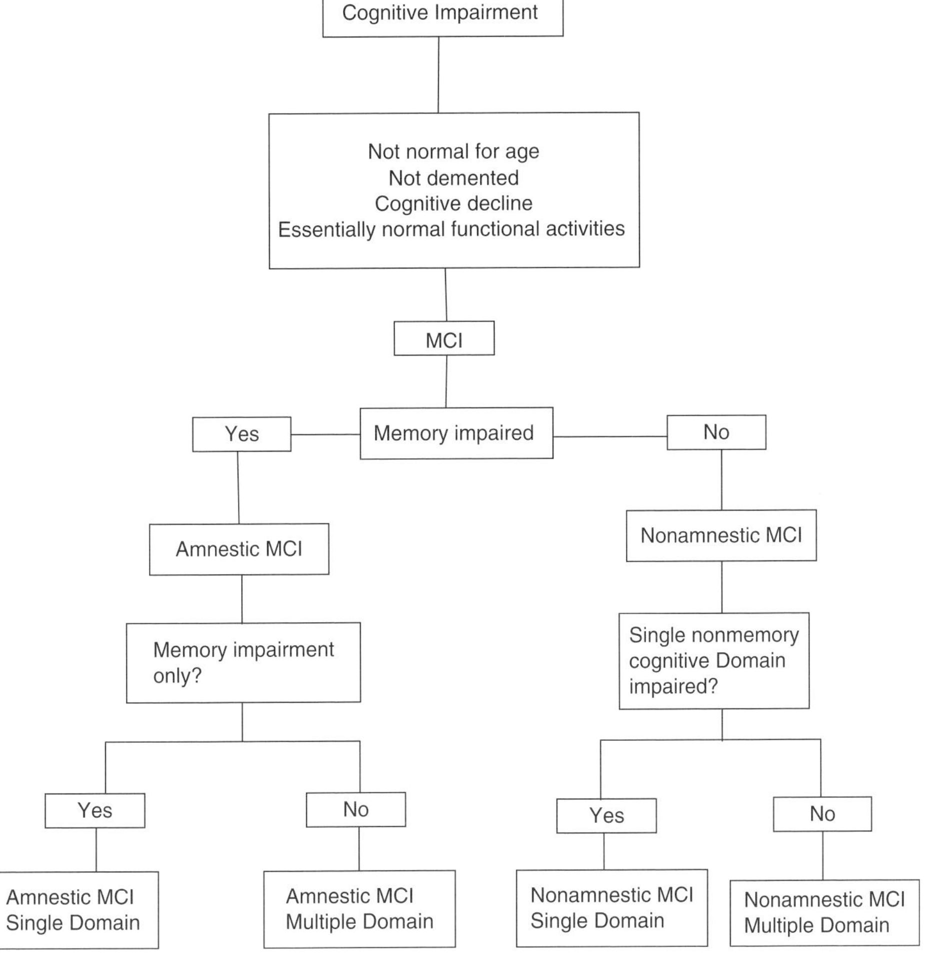

Figure 2.1 Algorithm for complete diagnosis for MCI. From Petersen [12,13].

defining MCI. Age-associated memory impairment and CIND are more broad in their categorization and have higher prevalence rates of nearly 20% [14,15] and 16·8% [16] respectively, while Petersen's criterion is narrow and rigid and has a prevalence of 3% [9]. Among the different types of MCI, a multicenter population study [17] found that the multiple cognitive deficits type (16%) was more prevalent as compared to the amnestic type (6%). Higher prevalence of md-MCI as compared to a-MCI has been confirmed by subsequent studies [18].

Clinical features, diagnosis, and prognosis of MCI

Mild cognitive impairment is characterized by impairment in cognitive domains that is intermediary between normal aging and dementia. While a-MCI is characterized by problems with memory, individuals with md-MCI are additionally impaired in other cognitive domains like activities of daily living and judgment. In the single non-memory MCI, there is mild impairment in executive function or visuospatial impairment other than memory. Individuals with MCI have subtle impairments in the conceptual knowledge of finance, cash transactions, bank statement management, and bill payment, and in overall financial capacity [19]. Mild cognitive impairment has been associated with impairment in motor coordination and balance leading to an increased risk of falling with subsequent soft-tissue injuries and fractures [20,21]. Cognitively impaired elderly without dementia have a greater mortality risk, hazard ratio of 1.7, as compared with cognitively unimpaired elderly [22]. Besides cognitive impairment, MCI has been consistently associated with behavioral problems similar to dementia. Apostolova and Cummings [23] conducted a meta-analysis of these symptoms and concluded that "neuropsychiatric symptoms in MCI are very common, occurring in 35–75% of patients." They noted that apathy, anxiety, depression, irritability, and agitation were among the most common behavioral symptoms while euphoria, hallucinations, disinhibition, and aberrant motor behavior were the least common. Additionally, the meta-analysis [24] also revealed that these neuropsychiatric symptoms were closely related to deterioration in cognition.

Neuropsychological tests and neuroimaging in MCI

Since the introduction of the neuropsychological dimension in the definition, a number of neuropsychological tests [25] have been identified as being useful in the detection of the early cognitive changes associated with MCI. In a longitudinal follow-up study, which has hence been confirmed [26], it was found that measures of memory, particularly delayed recall (with semantic cues), discriminated most accurately between subjects who subsequently developed AD (also identified as a predictor of conversion) and subjects who remained non-demented. Individuals with MCI have impairments in task-switching capacities that improve with practice [27], have impaired identification of "famous faces" [28], and have impaired facial emotion recognition [29–31]; all of which are intermediate between normal controls and AD. The Mini-Mental State Examination (MMSE) remains an excellent bedside screening test for cognitive impairment; combined with the clock-drawing test the diagnostic accuracy of the MMSE further increases. Another useful bedside complement for the MMSE is the Montreal Cognitive Assessment. Questionnaires such as the IQCODE (Informant Questionnaire on Cognitive Decline in the Elderly), which are based on reports of cognitive decline by the informants, can also be useful tools in diagnosing MCI [32].

Neuropathological data indicate the presence of neuritic plaques and neurofibrillary tangles in medial temporal (entorhinal, perirhinal, and hippocampal) regions akin to a progressive AD pathology [33]. Neuro Fibrillary tangles have also been reported in the nucleus basalis of Meynert similar to normal aging but more severe. This has been correlated with structural imaging (MRI) studies [34] that have noted atrophy in the entorhinal cortex and reductions in the temporal and parietal association cortices. Positron emission tomography and arterial spin MR imaging [35] studies have confirmed hypometabolism in parietotemporal, hippocampal, and the posterior cingulate gyrus regions. Magnetic resonance spectroscopy studies have demonstrated increased myoinositol/creatinine in the posterior cingulate gyrus and white matter of MCI patients confirming that the pathology in MCI is intermediate between MCI and aging. Amyloid markers such as the positron-emitting [11C]benzothiazole derivative known as Pittsburgh compound-B (PIB) and FDDNP [36] have also demonstrated diffuse amyloid pathology in the medial temporal regions. Mild cognitive impairment subjects have reduced medial temporal activations (hippocampus) on memory processing tasks [37,38]. A recent fMRI study [39] identified differences in memory encoding and retrieval; reductions in the activation of the frontal regions during encoding and of both frontal lobes and hippocampus during retrieval were noted. Impaired integrity of association tracts between a number of remote cortices has been reported by Bai *et al.* [40]; the FA (fractional anisotropy) values in some tracts were negatively correlated with performance on cognitive tests. Recent work by Popp *et al.* [41] indicates towards inflammatory processes that may contribute to the development and progression of the illness. They observed that levels of macrophage migration inhibitory factor may be elevated in the cerebrospinal fluid (CSF) of individuals with MCI.

MCI as a predictor of dementia

A wide variation in rates of conversion has been reported ranging from 6% to 25% per annum depending on the study criteria. One of the earliest outcome studies is the Mayo Clinic's longitudinal study of aging and dementia [42]. Subjects with MCI were followed up at four- and six-year intervals; conversion rates were 12% and 80% respectively. Seventy percent to 80% of patients with MCI and 50% of patients at the end of two years and five years respectively remained non-demented. Since then a number of studies have been carried out, including both clinic-based and population-based samples using varied criteria (Table 2.1). Population-based studies have confirmed that up to 44% of patients [55] with MCI return to normal cognitive functioning a year later, suggesting lack of temporal stability. Clinic-based studies have shown higher conversion rates as compared to population-based studies demonstrating an

Table 2.1 List of the major studies that have examined annual conversion rates of various definitions of MCI to dementia

	Source	Criteria	Annual conversion rate (% per year)	Comments
Mayo [9,42]	Memory disorders clinic	Memory loss	12	APOE4 allele carriers have a rapid progression
Toronto [43]	Family practice	Memory loss	14	Delayed recall and index of mental control
Seattle [44]	Health Maintenance Organization	Isolated memory loss	12	No single test can predict conversion
NYU [45]	Dementia clinic	GDS 3	25	
Harvard [46]	Community	CDR 0.5	6	
France [47]		MCI and AACD	11.1	MCI-unstable; AACD has higher conversion
PAQUID [48]	Community	Objective memory impairment	8.3	> 40% revert to normal
Religious Order study [49]	Catholic clergy	Multiple cognitive domains	7.7	
Rush Memory and Aging Project [50]	Memory disorders clinic	Multiple cognitive domains	10	
Kungsholmen Project [51,52]	Community	CIND	10	- 25% normal conversion irrespective of severity

				- neuropsychiatric- and frailty-related factors may affect cognition
REAL.FR cohort [53]	Community	CDR 0.5	32.5	Diagnostic stability of CDR
Bologna [54]	Memory disorders clinic	MCI (revised), CDR 0.5	a-MCI – 18.4, na-MCI – 19.7, md-MCI – 25.1 per 100 person-year	Higher HDL and lower folate levels may influence conversion

HDL, high-density lipoprotein; na-MCI, non-amnestic MCI.

underlying bias of superior cognitive evaluation and improved screening in clinic-based samples. Additionally, narrow criteria such as Petersen's have higher conversion rates as compared to AAMI and CIND. On an average, Reisberg *et al.* [56] have suggested a seven-year lag period to conversion to dementia from MCI.

It has been suggested that a-MCI preferentially progresses to Alzheimer's dementia, md-MCI may progress to AD or vascular dementia or often qualifies as normal aging while the single non-memory domain usually progresses to non-Alzheimer-type dementia. Multiple-domain MCI has also been associated with higher prevalence of arterial hypertension, and vascular lesions at brain imaging conforming to definitions of vascular MCI. A more recent study [57] has however questioned this differential progression, suggesting "partial" conformity.

Predictors of conversion

1. Poor performance on delayed recall, particularly cued recall, has been recognized as an important clinical predictor of conversion. Additionally, performance on MMSE, BVRT (visual working memory), and Isaacs Set Test (involving semantic verbal fluency) [58], baseline memory and executive performance [59] and low olfactory identification scores on the University of Pennsylvania Smell Identification Test [60] have been identified as notable predictors.
2. The presence of comorbid depression with poor response to antidepressants can double the risk of developing dementia [61]. The presence of other behavioral symptoms such as anxiety also increases the conversion rate [62].
3. Percent ventricular volume on MRI [63], baseline hippocampal atrophy [64], parietal asymmetry on PET [65], high CSF tau–cerebral blood Flow index [66], atrophy in the medial occipitotemporal cortex especially the combined middle and inferior temporal gyri [67], and parahippocampal and inferior temporal hypoperfusion [68] can be important imaging indices in identifying converters. Yuan *et al.* [69] provide a very useful meta-analysis comparing the various non-invasive imaging modalities as predictors of rapid conversion and conclude that FDG PET may have a better predictive accuracy as compared to SPECT or MRI.
4. Elevated levels of isoprostane 8, 12-iso-iPF_2-VI [70], presence of tau protein, hyperphosphorylated tau protein, amyloid β 42 protein [71,72], and ratio of plasma A_42/40[73,74] are emerging as sensitive biomarkers in the prediction of conversion to AD. A recent study [75] has indicated that accumulation of toxic substances such as homocysteine may also help predict conversion. Xu *et al.* [76] have suggested that increased levels of plasma fibrinogen/hyperfibrinogenemia may increase risk of dementia.
5. Finally, family history of AD and the presence of APOE4 genotype in subjects with MCI [77] have also been demonstrated to be significant predictors of conversion. Barabash *et al.* [78] have identified potential modifier genes and suggested that polymorphisms in α-1-antichymotrypsin

(ACT) may hasten while polymorphisms in CHRNA7 may attenuate the time of progression to AD.

Transcultural perspectives

In the setting of non-western cultures, accurately identifying persons with MCI and differentiating this from dementia can be a challenging task. For example in a recent clinic-based study (E. S. Krishnamoorthy, unpublished data) conducted in Chennai, people diagnosed by an experienced clinical neurologist as having MCI were found to have MMSE scores that ranged from 16 to 27. Assuming that the clinical impression was the gold standard, the problem may well have been with the standardization of MMSE. Yet, the version of the MMSE that was in use had been adapted from the validated Hindi MMSE [79] and had been previously used in large-scale screening of community-living elderly with consistent results [80]. Difficulties in differentiating MCI from dementia in these cultures also stem from socio-cultural attitudes and beliefs surrounding aging. One criticism of Western diagnostic criteria is that they are heavily weighted towards disability, relevant in highly individualistic societies, where independence has great value. Studies [80] show that when disability as a diagnostic criterion is removed, the prevalence of dementia is more or less equal across cultures. Further, clinical experience suggests that impairment of activities of daily living, while being an appropriate focus in the west, where many elderly people live alone and are relatively unsupported, is less relevant in the developing nation setting. Here, complex activities of daily living such as cooking of food, shopping, managing one's finances are often assumed, quite naturally, by the younger generation. As a consequence, disability in the older person becomes apparent and is reported only when even simple activities of daily living are impaired. There may thus be a need to conceptually examine and validate MCI as a concept in non-western cultures and more traditional societies in the Western world. The clinical impression in countries like India is that the spectrum of cognitive impairment is wider and more diffuse and therefore diagnostic accuracy becomes more difficult. Only significant cognitive impairment that impairs complex activities of daily living can be diagnosed easily and with accuracy. Table 2.2 provides a list of cross-sectional and longitudinal studies that have examined prevalence of MCI, neuropsychiatric symptoms in MCI and rates of conversion to dementia in non-Europe, non-US regions.

Management of MCI

Memory and other cognitive problems can have a tremendous impact on both the patients as well as their family members. The dementia drugs (cholinesterase inhibitors for example) are under active trials for MCI at present and the jury is still out about their utility with regard to either reversing MCI or indeed delaying the onset of conversion to dementia. In the absence of definitive pharmacotherapy, a number of other methods are in vogue and are briefly described here.

1. Acetylcholinesterase inhibitors such as donepezil, rivastigmine, and galantamine have not demonstrated long-term efficacy [94]. The Memory Impairment Study [95] suggested that donepezil maybe efficacious

Table 2.2 Select epidemiological studies that have examined prevalence of MCI, neuropsychiatric symptoms in MCI and progression to dementia in non-US, non-Europe regions

Region/ Country	Authors	Description	Age (average) yrs	Result	Comments
India					
	Banerjee *et al.* [81]	Longitudinal community-based	> 50	Instability of diagnosis as well as progression of MCI	Only eight participants had MCI
	Das *et al.* [82]	Cross-sectional community-based	> 50	Prevalence: MCI – 14.89%; a-MCI – 6.04%; md-MCI – 8.85%	
Australia					
PATH THROUGH LIFE study	Kumar *et al.* [83]	Cross-sectional community-based	60–64	Prevalence of MCI: 13.7%	Variation among various diagnostic criteria of AACD, MCI, AAMI
	Anstey *et al.* [84]	4-year follow up community-based		Prevalence of MCI: 4.2%	No conversion to dementia noted. AACD was a more stable diagnosis
Argentina	Mías *et al.* [85]	Cross-sectional	64.24	Prevalence: 9.1% – a-MCI; 4.5% – md-MCI	
China					
	Qiu *et al.* [86]	Cross-sectional community-based	> 55	Prevalence of MCI: 2.4%	
	Xiao *et al.* [87]	Longitudinal F/U of 47 MCI		13 developed dementia	Neuropsychological Battery of Cognitive Assessment Instruments developed by World Health Organization

					(WHO BCAI) had a 90% predictive accuracy rate
	Xu *et al.* [88]	Longitudinal, clinic-based, cross-cultural (Chinese vs. Americans)			Chinese subjects less likely (18.5%) to progress to Alzheimer's dementia as compared to Americans (47.9%)
Japan					
Nakayama Study	Ikeda and Shigenobu [89]	Community-based	> 65	Prevalence of MCI: 5.3%	
	Ishikawa *et al.* [90]	Longitudinal study F/U of Nakayama		Annual conversion rate to AD – 8.5% per 100 person-year	MMI/ND and not MCI
Tajiri Project	Meguro *et al.* [91]	Community-based	> 65	Prevalence of: MCI: 4.9%	Memory complaints not very useful. CDR 0.5 more accurate
Korea	Lee *et al.* [92]	Clinic-based cross-sectional evaluation of NPS	72.26	41.2% had NPS	No differences in NPS among different types of MCI Depression was the most commonly reported NPS
Taiwan	Wang *et al.* [93]	Clinic-based longitudinal evaluation of predictors of dementia		Cognitive performance had a greater influence on conversion as compared to hippocampal atrophy	APOE4 is associated with poorer cognitive performance and smaller hippocampi, but is not a predictor of conversion to dementia

F/u, follow-up; MMI/ND, mild memory impairment/No dementia; NPS, Neuropsychiatric symptoms.

in improving symptoms in the first year; however these benefits peter off over a longer term.

2. Control of cardiovascular risk factors particularly isolated systolic hypertension [26], treatment of comorbid conditions such as depression and medical conditions such as hypothyroidism and phasing out anticholinergic medications currently form the mainstay of intervention in MCI.
3. One promising therapy stems from the possible neuroprotective effects of calcium channel blockers. In a recent 20-month follow-up study, Hanyu *et al.* [96] noted that nilvadipine as against amlodipine was effective in slowing progression to MCI. However, this study examined a small sample of 15 patients and needs to be confirmed with larger randomized controlled tirals.
4. Nootropics (like piracetam and aniracetam) [97] have been shown to be active on different components of memory (notably recall) and also on other intellectual functions such as attention, concentration, and language. Preliminary results with phosphatidylserine [98] and ginkgo biloba extract [99] have been promising. Medications targeted at the secondary disease mechanisms can help in slowing down the neurodegenerative cascade and can thus help in delaying the onset of severe mental handicap. This category includes antioxidants such as vitamin E, anti-inflammatory drugs, and estrogen and has been useful in Alzheimer's dementia; however, their efficacy in MCI remains largely dubious.
5. Cognitive intervention measures such as cognitive stimulation, cognitive training, and cognitive rehabilitation have been suggested as possible interventions [100], although their efficacy has not been definitively established. Cognitive behavior therapy can be used to teach individuals with MCI to live with their difficulties and not be ashamed of them. Identifying the preserved areas of strength besides the areas of decline can prove useful in planning therapeutic strategies. Therapy should also be targeted towards building up the patients' self-esteem. The patient with MCI will need constant reassurance concerning the decline of his/her cognitive abilities. Individual counseling, helping the individual cope with the uncertainty of prognosis and increased mortality risks, along with family support should also be planned. A recent study [101] has noted promising improvements in cognition, occupational performance, and quality of life with goal-oriented rehabilitation therapy (similar to therapy employed for traumatic brain injury) comprising training in compensatory techniques, mind-mapping, and occupational therapy. Besides rehabilitation measures, individuals can also be encouraged to finalize important financial and legal decisions.
6. Finally, as in dementia and other chronic illnesses, caregivers of individuals with MCI can experience tremendous stress and need to be appropriately psychoeducated regarding the prognosis of the disorder and taught methods of reducing stress and avoiding burnout.

It is of importance that the patient and his/her family realize that the diagnosis of MCI does not necessarily imply the onset of dementia. Rehabilitation programs thus need to be tailored to suit the specific strengths, deficits, and needs of the individual. It has been suggested that medications such as anticholinesterase inhibitors can be tried on an individual basis. Individuals leading an active life with cognitive impairment impeding their daily functioning may benefit from medications as against individuals leading retired lives with minimal functional impairment. Currently, the mainstay of management however continues to be risk modification and lifestyle management.

Future directions

A multitude of criticisms have been raised regarding the current accepted criteria for MCI [11]. It has been suggested that the diagnosis of cognitive impairment should be tailored to account for age and premorbid capacity. Attenuation of cognitive function is an accompaniment of normal aging and is often determined by overall intellectual workouts performed by individuals. Additionally, it has been noted that while individuals may have functional impairment in their daily activities, they may perform adequately on neuropsychological tests, thereby missing the diagnosis of MCI; in other words, the "ecological validity" of the tests needs to be operationalized. Additionally, newer modalities of imaging including amyloid markers such as FDDNP and identification of genetic markers may enhance prediction of conversion.

The role of cognitive reserve (CR) [102] in the discrepancy between neuropathology and clinical manifestations of cognitive impairments including MCI is rapidly gaining importance. Cognitive reserve has been defined as hypothesized capacity of an adult brain to cope with brain pathology in order to minimize symptomatology. While the structural/anatomical CR refers to a threshold below which individuals remain asymptomatic, functional CR identifies alternate neural networks that can be recruited as compensation. This in turn reflects upon the individuals' educational/occupational attainment, premorbid intelligence quotient, leisure activities, and cognitive and mental stimulating activities. Thus enhancement of CR to potentiate compensation can form an important primary preventive measure and may explain the usefulness of cognitive retraining in MCI.

Is there a pre-MCI stage? – subjective cognitive impairment

Reisberg and Gauthier [103] have proposed that a prodromal stage to MCI exists that is characterized by subjective memory complaints – subjective cognitive impairment. This has been further described as GDS stage 2 – no neurological deficits with subjective memory impairment. These individuals have been identified as having three times greater risk of converting to dementia. Reisberg and Gauthier have further suggested that there may be a lag period of 15 years in individuals with SCI before they develop MCI [103]. Subjective cognitive impairment has also been associated with EEG changes in the form of increasing theta waves, reductions in parietotemporal and parahippocampal metabolism on PET, and hippocampal and gray matter changes on MRI consistent with progressive cognitive impairment. However, it has also been noted that SCI may be complicated by the presence of depression, with approximately twice the number of individuals developing major depression as compared to individuals without memory complaints. A recent study identified that impairment of olfaction is a predictor of MCI [104]! With MCI shrouded in the clouds of an existential dilemma, currently, SCI – a pre-MCI stage – is indeed only hypothetical.

Conclusion

What is clear from reviewing the literature is that each of the above descriptions has succeeded in capturing just one part of this wide interface, hence the appearance with time of newer descriptions that attempt to improve on the previous one and succeed in part. Mild cognitive impairment is the latest among these developments, and while at face value it appears comprehensive, it is not without pitfalls. Consider for example the criteria, which explicitly state "no impact on activities of daily living (ADL)"; yet the descriptions and typology indicate a clear impact on ADL, at least as the disorder progresses. What is abundantly clear also is that not all patients who enter this interface progress to dementia. While premature death may ensure that some do not, there clearly are others who may exist as long as five years without demonstrating significant progression. It is also interesting that the development of cerebral pathology may to some extent predicate such progression. However, with the predictors and mechanisms of cognitive decline being understood only in part, it is not entirely clear who among us will progress to dementia.

Mild cognitive impairment is currently "stuck between the proverbial deep blue sea and the devil" arising from epidemiological evidence and specialist neurological data. Thus while there are experts petitioning for the recognition of MCI in the Diagnostic and Statistical Manual of Mental Disorders, fifth edition (DSM-V) [105], several others query the existence of MCI as a clinical entity. Diagnosing MCI is also fraught with clinical and ethical concerns. On the one hand, MCI probably provides the earliest and thereby the best stage for initiating anti-dementia measures. On the other, it must be acknowledged that not all individuals with MCI progress to dementia and such a diagnosis may be counterproductive for people who are otherwise well integrated. With the subdivisions of MCI remaining poorly accepted, and the prospect of definitive treatment distant, diagnosis and the management of such a patient once diagnosed remains a challenge and cause for trepidation even for the experienced and accomplished clinician.

Finally, the transcultural issues identified herein highlight the importance of a transcultural approach to developing concepts surrounding cognitive impairment. Currently the top-down approach that is prevalent results in predominantly western concepts being applied in non-western cultures. Cognitive impairment being a spectrum of conditions from physiological to pathological necessitates a bottom-up approach in order to understand better and determine precisely its disability and handicap.

Indeed, as in the title of this book a global approach to this important area is urgently required.

References

1. Kral VA. Senescent forgetfulness: benign and malignant. *Can Med Assoc J* 1962; **86**: 257–60.
2. Kral VA. Neuropsychiatric observations in an old people's home. Studies of memory dysfunction in senescence. *J Gerontol* 1958; **13**: 169–76.
3. Crook TH, Bartus RT, Ferris SH, *et al.* Age-associated memory impairment: Proposed diagnostic criteria and measures of clinical change – Report of a National Institute of Mental Health work group. *Dev Neuropsychol* 1986; **2**: 261–76.
4. Blackford RC, La Rue A. Criteria for diagnosing age-associated memory impairment: proposed improvements from the field. *Dev Neuropsychol* 1989; **5**: 295–306.
5. Levy R. Aging associated cognitive decline. *Int Psychogeriatr* 1994; **6**: 63–8
6. Ebly EM, Hogan DB, Parhad IM. Cognitive impairment in the non-demented elderly: results from the Canadian Study on Health and Aging. *Arch Neurol* 1995; **52**: 612–19.
7. Tierney MC, Herrmann F, Geslani D, Szalai J. Contribution of informant and patient ratings to the accuracy of the mini-mental State examination in predicting probable Alzheimer's disease. *J Am Geriatr Soc* 2003; **51**: 813–18.
8. Gauthier S, Reisberg B, Zaudig M, *et al.* Mild cognitive impairment. *Lancet* 2006; **367**; 1262–70.
9. Petersen RC, Smith GE, Waring SC, *et al.* Mild cognitive impairment. Clinical characterization and outcome. *Arch Neurol* 1999; **56**: 303–8.
10. Portet F, Ousset PJ, Visser PJ, *et al.* MCI working group of the European Consortium on Alzheimer's disease (EADC). Mild cognitive impairment (MCI) in medical practice: critical review of the concept and new diagnostic procedure. Report of the MCI working group of the European Consortium on Alzheimer's disease (EADC). *J Neurol Neurosurg Psychiatry* 2006; **77**: 714–18.
11. Nordlund A, Rolstad S, Hellström P, *et al.* The Goteborg MCI study: mild cognitive impairment is a heterogeneous condition. *J Neurol Neurosurg Psychiatry* 2005; **76**: 1485–90.
12. Petersen RC. Mild cognitive impairment as a diagnostic entity. *J Intern Med* 2004; **256**: 183–94.
13. Petersen RC. Mild cognitive impairment. *Continum* 2004; **10**: 9–28.
14. Ritchie K, Artero S, Touchon J. Classification criteria for mild cognitive impairment: a population-based validation study. *Neurology* 2001 **56**: 37–42.
15. Graham JE, Rockwood K, Beattie BL, *et al.* Prevalence and severity of cognitive impairment with and without dementia in an elderly population. *Lancet* 1997; **349**: 1793–6.
16. Goldman WP, Morris JC. Evidence that age-associated memory impairment is not a normal variant of aging. *Alzheimer Dis Assoc Disord* 2001; **15**: 72–9.
17. Lopez OL, Jagust WJ, DeKosky ST, *et al.* Prevalence and classification of mild cognitive impairment in the Cardiovascular Health Study Cognition Study: part 1. *Arch Neurol* 2003; **60**: 1385–9.
18. Zanetti M, Ballabio C, Abbate C, *et al.* Mild cognitive impairment subtypes and vascular dementia in community-dwelling elderly people: a 3-year follow-up study. *J Am Geriatr Soc* 2006; **54**: 580–6.

19. Griffith HR, Belue K, Sicola A, *et al.* Impaired financial abilities in mild cognitive impairment: a direct assessment approach. *Neurology* 2003; **60**: 449–57.

20. Mahoney J, Sager M, Dunnan NC, Thomson J. Risk of falls after hospital discharge. *J Am Geriatr Soc* 1994 **42**: 269–74.

21. Myers AH, Young Y, Langlois JA. Prevention of falls in elderly. *Bone* 1996; **18**(1 Suppl): 875–1015.

22. Frisoni GB, Fratiglioni L, Fastbom J, Viitanen M, Winblad B. Mortality in nondemented subjects with cognitive impairment: the influence of health-related factors. *Am J Epidemiol* 1999; **150**(10): 1031–44.

23. Apostolova LG, Cummings JL. Neuropsychiatric manifestations in mild cognitive impairment: a systematic review of the literature. *Dement Geriatr Cogn Disord* 2008; **25**: 115–26.

24. Palmer K, Berger AK, Monastero R, *et al.* Predictors of progression from mild cognitive impairment to Alzheimer disease. *Neurology* 2007; **68**(19): 1596–602.

25. Chen P, Ratcliff G, Belle SH, *et al.* Cognitive tests that best discriminate between presymptomatic AD and those who remain nondemented. *Neurology* 2000; **55**: 1847–53.

26. Gauthier S, Reisberg B, Zaudig M, *et al.* International Psychogeriatric Association Expert Conference on mild cognitive impairment. Mild cognitive impairment. *Lancet* 2006; **367**(9518): 1262–70.

27. Belleville S, Bherer L, Lepage E, Chertkow H, Gauthier S. Task switching capacities in persons with Alzheimer's disease and mild cognitive impairment. *Neuropsychologia* 2008; **46**: 2225–33.

28. Estévezfi-Gonzalez A, Garcí-Sánchez C, Otermín ABP, *et al.* Semantic knowledge of famous people in mild cognitive impairment and progression to alzheimer's disease. *Dement Geriatr Cogn Disord* 2004; **17**: 188–95.

29. Teng E, Lu PH, Cummings JL. Deficits in facial emotion processing in mild cognitive impairment. *Dement Geriatr Cogn Disord* 2007; **23**(4) 271–9.

30. Spoletini I, Marra C, Di Iulio F, *et al.* Facial emotion recognition deficit in amnestic mild cognitive impairment and Alzheimer disease. *Am J Geriatr Psychiatry* 2008; **16**(5): 389–98.

31. Weiss EM, Kohler CG, Vonbank J, *et al.* Impairment in emotion recognition abilities in patients with mild cognitive impairment, early and moderate Alzheimer disease compared with healthy comparison subjects. *Am J Geriatr Psychiatry* 2008; **16**(12): 974–80.

32. Petersen RC, Stevens JC, Ganguli M, *et al.* Practice parameter: early detection of dementia: mild cognitive impairment (evidence-based review). *Neurology* 2001; **56**: 1133–42.

33. Golomb J, Kluge A, Ferris SH. Mild cognitive impairment: historical development and summary of research. *Dialogues Clin Neurosci* 2004; **6**: 351–67.

34. Matsuda H The role of neuroimaging in mild cognitive impairment. *Neuropathology* 2007; **27**: 570–7.

35. Johnson NA, Jahng G, Weiner MW, *et al.* Pattern of cerebral hypoperfusion in Alzheimer disease and mild cognitive impairment measured with arterial spin-labeling MR Imaging: initial experience. *Radiology* 2005; **234**: 851–9.

36. Small GW, Kepe V, Ercoli LM, *et al.* PET of brain amyloid and tau in mild cognitive impairment. *N Engl J Med* 2006; **355**: 2652–63.

37. Machulda M, Ward H, Borowski B, *et al.* Comparison of memory fMRI response among

normal, MCI, and Alzheimer's patients. *Neurology* 2003; **61**: 500–6.

38. Johnson SC, Baxter LC, Susskind-Wilder L, *et al.* Hippocampal adaptation to face repetition in healthy elderly and mild cognitive impairment. *Neuropsychologia* 2004; **42**: 980–9.
39. Petrella JR, Krishnan S, Slavin MJ, Mild cognitive impairment: evaluation with 4-T functional MR imaging. *Radiology* 2006; **240**: 177–86.
40. Bai F, Zhang Z, Watson DR, *et al.* Abnormal integrity of association fiber tracts in amnestic mild cognitive impairment. *J Neurol Sci* 2009; **15** (278): 1–2.
41. Popp J, Bacher M, Kölsch H, *et al.* Macrophage migration inhibitory factor in mild cognitive impairment and Alzheimer's disease. *J Psychiatr Res* 2008; **43**(8): 749–53.
42. Petersen RC. Mild cognitive impairment: transition from aging to Alzheimer's disease. In: Iqbalk K, Sisodia SS, Winblad B, eds., *Alzheimer's Disease*. New York, Oxford University Press. 2003; 141–51.
43. Tierney MC, Szalai JP, Snow WG, *et al.* A prospective study of the clinical utility of ApoE genotype in the prediction of outcome in patients with memory impairment. *Neurology* 1996; **46**: 149–54.
44. Bowen J, Teri L, Kukull W, *et al.* Progression to dementia in patients with isolated memory loss. *Lancet* 1997; **349**: 763–5.
45. Flicker C, Ferris SH, Reisberg B. Mild cognitive impairment in the elderly: predictors of dementia. *Neurology* 1991; **41**: 1006–9.
46. Daly E, Zaitchik D, Copeland M, *et al.* Predicting conversion to Alzheimer disease using standardized clinical information. *Arch Neurol* 2000; **57**: 675–80.
47. Ritchie K, Artero S, Touchon J. Classification criteria for mild cognitive impairment: a population-based validation study. *Neurology* 2000; **56**: 37–42.
48. Larrieu S, Letenneur L, Orgogozo JM, *et al.* Incidence and outcome of mild cognitive impairment in a population-based prospective cohort. *Neurology* 2002; **59**: 1594–9.
49. Bennett DA, Wilson RS, Schneider JA, *et al.* Natural history of mild cognitive impairment in older persons. *Neurology* 2002; **59**: 198–205.
50. Boyle PA, Wilson RS, Aggarwal NT, Tang Y, Bennett DA. Mild cognitive impairment: risk of Alzheimer disease and rate of cognitive decline. *Neurology* 2006; **67**(3): 441–5.
51. Palmer K, Wang HX, Bäckman L, Winblad B, Fratiglioni L. Differential evolution of cognitive impairment in nondemented older persons: results from the Kungsholmen Project. *Am J Psychiatry* 2002; **159**(3): 436–42.
52. Monastero R, Palmer K, Qiu C, Winblad B, Fratiglioni L. Heterogeneity in risk factors for cognitive impairment, no dementia: population-based longitudinal study from the Kungsholmen Project. *Am J Geriatr Psychiatry* 2007; **15**(1): 60–9.
53. Nourhashémi F, Ousset PJ, Gillette-Guyonnet S, *et al.* A 2-year follow-up of 233 very mild (CDR 0.5) Alzheimer's disease patients (REAL.FR cohort). *Int J Geriatr Psychiatry* 2007; **23**(5): 460–5.
54. Maioli F, Coveri M, Pagni P, *et al.* Conversion of mild cognitive impairment to dementia in elderly subjects: a preliminary study in a memory and cognitive disorder unit. *Arch Gerontol Geriatr* 2007; **44**(Suppl 1): 233–41.
55. Ritchie K. Mild cognitive impairment: an epidemiological perspective. *Dialogues Clin Neurosci* 2004; **6**: 401–8.

56. Reisberg B, Ferris SH, Kluger A, *et al.* Mild cognitive impairment (MCI): a historical perspective. *Int Psychogeriatr* 2008; **20**(1): 18–31.

57. Busse A, Hensel A, Gühne U, Angermeyer MC, Riedel-Heller SG. Mild cognitive impairment: long-term course of four clinical subtypes. *Neurology* 2006; **67**(12): 2176–85.

58. Datrigues JF, Commenges D, Letenneur D, *et al.* Cognitive predictors of dementia in elderly community residents. *Neuroepidemiology* 1997; **16**: 29–39.

59. DeCarli C, Mungas D, Harvey D, *et al.* Memory impairment, but not cerebrovascular disease, predicts progression of MCI to dementia. *Neurology* 2004; **63**: 220–7.

60. Devanand DP, Michaels-Marston KS, Liu X, *et al.* Olfactory deficits in patients with mild cognitive impairment predict Alzheimer's disease at follow-up. *Am J Psychiatry* 2000; **157**: 1399–405.

61. Modrego PJ, Ferrández J. Depression in patients with mild cognitive impairment increases the risk of developing dementia of Alzheimer type: a prospective cohort study. *Arch Neurol* 2004; **61**: 1290–3.

62. Palmer K, Berger AK, Monastero R, *et al.* Predictors of progression from mild cognitive impairment to Alzheimer disease. *Neurology* 2007; **68**(19): 1596–602.

63. Adak S, Illouz K, Gorman W, Predicting the rate of cognitive decline in aging and early Alzheimer disease. *Neurology* 2004; **63**: 108–14.

64. Apostolova LG, Dutton RA, Dinov ID, *et al.* Conversion of mild cognitive impairment to Alzheimer disease predicted by hippocampal atrophy maps. *Arch Neurol* 2006; **63**: 693–9.

65. Small GW, Mazziotta JC, Collins MT, *et al.* Apolipoprotein E type 4 allele and cerebral glucose metabolism in relatives at risk for familial Alzheimer's disease. *JAMA* 1995; **273**: 942–7.

66. Okamura N, Arai H, Maruyama M, *et al.* Combined analysis of CSF tau levels and [^{123}I] Iodoamphetamine SPECT in mild cognitive impairment: implications for a novel predictor of Alzheimer's disease. *Am J Psychiatry* 2002; **159**: 474–6.

67. Convit A, de Asis J, de Leon MJ, *et al.* Atrophy of the medial occipitotemporal, inferior, and middle temporal gyri in non-demented elderly predict decline to Alzheimer's disease. *Neurobiol Aging* 2000; **21**(1): 19–26.

68. Caroli A, Testa C, Geroldi C, *et al.* Cerebral perfusion correlates of conversion to Alzheimer's disease in amnestic mild cognitive impairment. *J Neurol* 2007; **254**: 1698–707.

69. Yuan Y, Gu ZX, Wei WS. Fluorodeoxyglucose-positron-emission tomography, single-photon emission tomography, and structural MR imaging for prediction of rapid conversion to Alzheimer disease in patients with mild cognitive impairment: a meta-analysis. *Am J Neuroradiol* 2008; **30**(2): 404–10.

70. Praticò D, Clark CM, Liun F, Lee VY, Trojanowski JQ. Increase of brain oxidative stress in mild cognitive impairment. A possible predictor of Alzheimer disease. *Arch Neurol* 2002; **59**: 972–6.

71. Hampel H, Teipel SJ, Fuchsberger T, *et al.* Value of CSF beta amyloid-42 and tau as predictors of Alzheimer's disease in patients with mild cognitive impairment. *Mol Psychiatry* 2004; **9**: 705–10.

72. Maruyama M, Arai H, Sugita M, *et al.* Cerebrospinal fluid amyloid b *et al* (1–42) levels in the mild cognitive impairment stage of Alzheimer's disease. *Exp Neurol* 2001; **172**: 433–6.

73. Oijen V, Hofman A, Soares HD, Koudstaal PJ, Breteler MM. Plasma Abeta(1–40) and Abeta (1–42) and the risk of dementia: a prospective case-cohort study. *Lancet Neurol* 2006; **5**: 655–60.

74. Graff-Radford NR, Crook JE, Lucas J, *et al.* Association of low plasma Abeta42/Abeta40 ratios with increased imminent risk for mild cognitive impairment and Alzheimer disease. *Arch Neurol* 2007; **64**: 354–62.

75. Blasko I, Jellinger K, Kemmler G, *et al.* Conversion from cognitive health to mild cognitive impairment and Alzheimer's disease: prediction by plasma amyloid beta 42, medial temporal lobe atrophy and homocysteine. *Neurobiol Aging* 2008; **29**: 1–11.

76. Xu G, Zhang H, Zhang S, Fan X, Liu X. Plasma fibrinogen is associated with cognitive decline and risk for dementia in patients with mild cognitive impairment. *Int J Clin Pract* 2008; **62**(7): 1070–5.

77. Petersen RC, Smith GE, Ivnik RJ, *et al.* Apolipoprotein E status as a predictor of the development of Alzheimer's disease in memory-impaired individuals. *JAMA* 1995; **273**(16): 1274–8.

78. Barabash A, Marcos A, Ancín I, *et al.* APOE, ACT and CHRNA7 genes in the conversion from amnestic mild cognitive impairment to Alzheimer's disease. *Neurobiol Aging* 2009; **30**(8): 1254–64.

79. Ganguli M, Ratcliff G, Chandra V, *et al.* A Hindi version of the MMSE: the development of a cognitive screening instrument for a largely illiterate rural elderly population in India. *Int J Geriatr Psychiatry* 1995; **10**: 367–77.

80. Rodriguez JLL, Ferri CP, Acosta D, *et al.* for the 10/66 Dementia Research Group. Prevalence of dementia in Latin America, India, and China: a population-based cross-sectional survey. *Lancet* 2008; **372** (9637): 464–74

81. Banerjee TK, Mukherjee CS, Dutt A, Shekhar A, Hazra A. Cognitive dysfunction in an urban Indian population – some observations. *Neuroepidemiology* 2008; **31**(2): 109–14.

82. Das SK, Bose P, Biswas A, *et al.* An epidemiological study of mild cognitive impairment in Kolkata, India. *Neurology* 2007; **68**(23): 2019–26.

83. Kumar R, Dear KBG, Christensen H, *et al.* Prevalence of mild cognitive impairment in 60- to 64-year-old community-dwelling individuals: The Personality and Total Health through Life 60+ Study. *Dement Geriatr Cogn Disord* 2005; **19**: 67–74.

84. Anstey KJ, Cherbuin N, Christensen H, *et al.* Follow-up of mild cognitive impairment and related disorders over four years in adults in their sixties: the PATH Through Life Study. *Dement Geriatr Cogn Disord* 2008; **26**: 226–33.

85. Mías CD, Sassi M, Masih ME, Querejeta A, Krawchik R. [Mild cognitive impairment: a prevalence and sociodemographic factors study in the city of Córdoba, Argentina.] *Rev Neurol* 2007; **44**(12): 733–8.

86. Qiu CJ, Tang MN, Zhang W, *et al.* [The prevalence of mild cognitive impairment among residents aged 55 or over in Chengdu area.] *Zhonghua Liu Xing Bing Xue Za Zhi* 2003; **24**(12): 1104–7.

87. Xiao SF, Xue HB, Li GJ, *et al.* [Outcome and cognitive changes of mild cognitive impairment in the elderly: a follow-up study of 47 cases.] *Zhonghua Yi Xue Za Zhi* 2006; **86**(21): 1441–6.

88. Xu G, Meyer JS, Huang Y, *et al.* Cross-cultural comparison of mild cognitive impairment between China and USA. *Curr Alzheimer Res* 2004; **1**(1): 55–61.

89. Ikeda M, Shigenobu K. [The prevalence of mild cognitive impairment (MCI) among the community-dwelling elderly: findings from the

2nd Nakayama study.] *Seishin Shinkeigaku Zasshi* 2003; **105**(4): 381–6

90. Ishikawa T, Ikeda M, Matsumoto N, *et al.* A longitudinal study regarding conversion from mild memory impairment to dementia in a Japanese community. *Int J Geriatr Psychiatry* 2006; **21**: 134–9.
91. Meguro K, Ishii H, Yamaguchi S, *et al.* Prevalence and cognitive performances of clinical dementia rating 0.5 and mild cognitive impairment in Japan. The Tajiri project. *Alzheimer Dis Assoc Disord* 2004; **18**(1): 3–10.
92. Lee KS, Cho H, Hong CH, Kim DG, Oh BH. Differences in neuropsychiatric symptoms according to mild cognitive impairment subtypes in the community. *Dement Geriatr Cogn Disord* 2008; **26**: 212–17.
93. Wang PN, Lirng JF, Lin KN, Chang FC, Liu HC. Prediction of Alzheimer's disease in mild cognitive impairment: a prospective study in Taiwan. *Neurobiol Aging* 2006; **27**: 1797–806.
94. Raschetti R, Albanese E, Vanacore N, Maggini M. Cholinesterase inhibitors in mild cognitive impairment: a systematic review of randomized trials. *PLoS Med* 2007; **4**(11): e338.
95. Petersen RC, Thomas RG, Grundman M, *et al.* Alzheimer's Disease Cooperative Study Group. Vitamin E and donepezil for the treatment of mild cognitive impairment. *N Engl J Med* 2005; **352**: 2379–88.
96. Hanyu H, Hirao K, Shimizu S, *et al.* Nilvadipine prevents cognitive decline of patients with mild cognitive impairment. *Int J Geriatr Psychiatry* 2007; **22**: 1264–6.
97. Pasquier F. Minimal cognitive impairment. In: Gauthier S, Cummings JL, eds. *Alzheimer's Disease and related Disorders Annual.* London, Martin Dunitz Ltd. 2000; 135–54.
98. Crook TH, Tinklenberg J, Yesavage J, *et al.* Effects of phosphatidylserine in age-associated memory impairment. *Neurology* 1991; **41**(5): 644–9.
99. Brautigam MRH, Blommart FA, Varleye G, *et al.* Treatment of age-related memory complaints with gingko biloba extract, a randomized double-blind placebo-controlled study. *Phytomedicine* 1998; **5**: 425–34.
100. Belleville S. Cognitive training for persons with mild cognitive impairment. *Int Psychogeriatr* 2008; **20**(1): 57–66.
101. Londos E, Boschian K, Lindén A, *et al.* Effects of a goal-oriented rehabilitation program in mild cognitive impairment: a pilot study. *Am J Alzheimers Dis Other Dement* 2008; **23**(2): 177–83.
102. Solé-Padullés C, Bartrés-Faz D, Junqué C, *et al.* Brain structure and function related to cognitive reserve variables in normal aging, mild cognitive impairment and Alzheimer's disease. *Neurobiol Aging* 2009; **30**(7): 1114–24.
103. Reisberg B, Gauthier S. Current evidence for subjective cognitive impairment (SCI) as the pre-mild cognitive impairment (MCI) stage of subsequently manifest Alzheimer's disease. *Int Psychogeriatr* 2008; **20**(1): 1–16.
104. Wilson RS, Schneider JA, Arnold SE, *et al.* Olfactory identification and incidence of mild cognitive impairment in older age. *Arch Gen Psychiatry* 2007; **64**(7): 802–8.
105. Petersen RC, O'Brien J. Mild cognitive impairment should be considered for DSM-V. *J Geriatr Psychiatry Neurol* 2006; **19**: 147–54.

Chapter 3

Alzheimer's disease: the African American story

Hugh Hendrie

Introduction

African Americans have historically been underrepresented in research studies into Alzheimer's disease (AD) and other dementias in the United States [1]. However, over the past decade there have been an increasing number of clinical and epidemiological studies in dementia that have included significant numbers of African Americans and have increased our knowledge of the nature and extent of the disease in this population.

Incidence of dementia and AD in African Americans

There are now several large cohort, population-based studies reporting on the incidence of dementia and AD in elderly African Americans. Two of these studies, which involve multiracial comparisons, the Chicago Study on Health and Aging and the Northern Manhattan Study, have reported higher incidence rates for African Americans as compared to whites. The age specific incidence rates for AD in African Americans in these two studies are similar (Chicago 65–74 1.79%, 75–84 6.06%, 85+ 12.72%, North Manhattan 65–74 1.7%, 75–84 4.4%, 85+ 11.4%) [2,3]. These rates are also similar but somewhat higher than the incidence rates reported from African Americans from the Indianapolis–Ibadan dementia project. (65–74 1.38%, 75–84 3.29%, 85+ 7.07) [4].

When the Indianapolis incidence rates for AD and dementia are compared to a meta-analysis, which included published incidence rates from other populations, the rates for African Americans are at the higher end of reported rates from other studies [5]. Not all studies agree, however. A study of African American and White populations in the Piedmont area of North Carolina [6], concluded that 3-year incidence rates of dementia were similar between races. In the Cardiovascular Health Study, the incidence rates for dementia in African Americans were only marginally

Dementia: A Global Approach, ed. Ennapadam S. Krishnamoorthy, Martin J. Prince, and Jeffrey L. Cummings. Published by Cambridge University Press.

higher than those for Whites after adjusting for education [7].

The role of education in risk for AD in African Americans

Low education is one of the most consistently reported risk factors for AD, dementia, and cognitive decline in all populations including African Americans. Education also influences scores in neuropsychological testing and differentially so for African Americans [8].

However, Manly and her colleagues [9] have concluded that education, at least as recorded by grade level, is an inadequate measurement of educational experience in African Americans because of the marked discrepancies between the quality of education in regions of the country as a residue of racial discriminatory policies. They have proposed that reading levels are a better measurement of educational attainment in African Americans and that adjusting for reading levels attenuates differences in neuropsychological test performance between African Americans and Whites.

In the study of African Americans living in Indianapolis, both low education and rural residence in childhood were risk factors for AD. There was a strong interaction between these factors however such that a combination of low education and rural residence mostly in the southern states of America increased the risk of developing AD sixfold as compared to higher-educated urban resident groups. The authors concluded that it is possible that low education by itself is not a major risk factor for AD but rather is a marker for other accompanying deleterious socioeconomic or environmental influences in childhood [10].

The genetics of AD in African Americans

There appears to be little doubt that, as in other populations, genetic factors play a major role in the etiology of late-onset AD in African Americans [11]. One major genetic risk factor in most populations is the possession of the e4 allele of APOE. Yet, the reported association of this allele with AD in African Americans is inconsistent. The Chicago-and North Manhattan-based studies report weak (i.e., only in persons with the e44 genotype) or no relationship in African Americans [2,12], whereas a robust relationship between the e4 allele and AD is reported from the MIRAGE study [13], and for African Americans living in Indianapolis [14]. The reasons for these discrepancies are unclear. It may be related to interactions between the e4 allele and other biological factors which differ between the populations (e.g., lipids) [15]. It may be the result of other genes which affect both AD risk and APOE gene expression and may differ between African Americans [14]. It is noteworthy that no association between APOEe4 and AD has been found in the Yoruba [16].

Other risk factors

There is now considerable evidence that vascular risk factors also increase the risk for AD. One of the most striking features of the Indianapolis–Ibadan comparative study is that not only is AD less common in Yoruba than in African Americans but so also are vascular diseases such as diabetes and hypertension [17]. African Americans are at higher risk for these diseases than White Americans. It has been proposed that the differences in rates of vascular illness may account for the higher rates of AD in African Americans. However, this explanation remains unproven at this time [3].

Conclusion

Dementia and AD is at least as common if not more common in African Americans as in other groups in United States. Hopefully the newer studies will provide some clues which will assist in the management and prevention of this devastating disease in the future.

References

1. Allery AJ, Aranda MP, Dilworth-Anderson P, *et al.* Alzheimer's disease and communities of color: In: Whitefield KE, ed. *Closing the Gap*: Improving the Health of Minority Elders in the New Millenium. Washington DC, Gerontological Society of America. 2004: 81–6.
2. Evans DA, Bennett DA, Wilson RS, *et al.* Incidence of Alzheimer disease in a biracial urban community: relation to apolipoprotein E allele status. *Arch Neurol* 2003; **60**(2): 185–9.
3. Tang MX, Cross P, Andrews H, *et al.* Incidence of AD in African-Americans, Caribbean Hispanics, and Caucasians in northern Manhattan. *Neurology* 2001; **56**(1): 49–56.
4. Hendrie HC, Ogunniyi A, Hall KS, *et al.* Incidence of dementia and Alzheimer disease in 2 communities: Yoruba residing in Ibadan, Nigeria, and African Americans residing in Indianapolis, Indiana. *JAMA* 2001; **285**(6): 739–47.
5. Gao S, Hendrie HC, Hall KS, Hui S. The relationships between age, sex, and the incidence of dementia and Alzheimer disease: a meta-analysis. *Arch Gen Psychiatry* 1998; **55**(9): 809–15.
6. Fillenbaum GG, Heyman A, Huber MS, *et al.* The prevalence and 3-year incidence of dementia in older Black and White community residents. *J Clin Epidemiol* 1998; **51**(7): 587–95.
7. Fitzpatrick AL, Kuller LH, Ives DG, *et al.* Incidence and prevalence of dementia in the Cardiovascular Health Study. *J Am Geriatr Soc* 2004; **52**(2): 195–204.
8. Hendrie HC, Albert MS, Butters MA, *et al.* The NIH Cognitive and Emotional Health Project: Report of the Critical Evaluation Study Committee. *Alzheimers Dement* 2006; **2**(1): 12–32.
9. Manly JJ, Jacobs DM, Touradji P, Small SA, Stern Y. Reading level attenuates differences in neuropsychological test performance between African American and White elders. *J Int Neuropsychol Soc* 2002; **8**(3): 341–8.
10. Hall KS, Gao S, Unverzagt FW, Hendrie HC. Low education and childhood rural residence: risk for Alzheimer's disease in African Americans. *Neurology* 2000; **54**(1): 95–9.
11. Green RC, Cupples LA, Go R, *et al.* Risk of dementia among white and African American relatives of patients with Alzheimer disease. *JAMA* 2002; **287**(3): 329–36.
12. Tang MX, Stern Y, Marder K, *et al.* The APOE-epsilon4 allele and the risk of Alzheimer disease among African Americans, whites, and Hispanics. *JAMA* 1998; **279**(10): 751–5.
13. Graff-Radford NR, Green RC, *et al.* Association between apolipoprotein E genotype and Alzheimer disease in African American subjects. *Arch Neurol* 2002; **59**(4): 594–600.

14. Murrell JR, Price B, Lane KA, *et al.* Association of apolipoprotein E genotype and Alzheimer disease in African Americans. *Arch Neurol* 2006; **63**(3): 431–4.

15. Hall K, Murrell J, Ogunniyi A, *et al.* Cholesterol, APOE genotype, and Alzheimer disease: an epidemiologic study of Nigerian Yoruba. *Neurology* 2006; **66**(2): 223–7.

16. Gureje O, Ogunniyi A, Baiyewu O, *et al.* APOE epsilon4 is not associated with Alzheimer's disease in elderly Nigerians. *Ann Neurol* 2006; **59**(1): 182–5.

17. Hendrie HC, Murrell J, Gao S, *et al.* International studies in dementia with particular emphasis on populations of African origin. *Alzheimer Dis Assoc Disord* 2006; **20**(3 Suppl 2): S42–6.

Vascular cognitive impairment

The syndrome of vascular cognitive impairment: current concepts

J. V. Bowler

Introduction

Vascular cognitive impairment (VCI) [1] has replaced the older concept of vascular dementia (VaD). It refers to cognitive impairment of any degree of severity arising from cerebrovascular disease of any kind and avoids the considerable limitations contained with the concept of VaD. These limitations arose because the principal definitions of VaD, contained within the *International Classification of Diseases*, tenth revision (ICD-10) [2] and the *Diagnostic and Statistical Manual of Mental Disorders*, fourth edition (DSM-IV) [3], are based on Alzheimer's disease (AD) and consequently emphasize memory loss and usually the progression and irreversibility of the cognitive decline, none of which are necessarily the case in VCI.

These basic definitions were operationalized in the NINDS-AIREN criteria [4] and the California criteria [5] but neither has met universal acceptance or been validated. Furthermore, they are difficult to apply consistently and produce very different results [6]. Their use in new work is not recommended but the NINDS-AIREN criteria in particular have been used in much of the published work available to date, even though they were developed with a view to epidemiological convenience rather than to clinical accuracy. A description of the limitations of these criteria forms a good basis for understanding the concept of VCI and allows interpretation of data derived using them.

Pattern of cognitive deficit in vascular dementia

The mesial temporal lobes are affected early in AD but not in VCI. A diagnostic paradigm based on early memory loss is consequently inappropriate and will fail to identify many cases of VCI. Data derived from those with cognitive impairment due to cerebrovascular

Dementia: A Global Approach, ed. Ennapadam S. Krishnamoorthy, Martin J. Prince, and Jeffrey L. Cummings. Published by Cambridge University Press.

disease who have not been preselected for having an amnestic syndrome reveal a predominating theme of a primarily subcortical dementia with early impairment of frontal lobe function. Memory impairment is usual but is often not preeminent.

The presence of "patchy" or unequal cognitive deficits is a requirement for a diagnosis of VaD in ICD-10 but this pattern of cognitive loss is only to be expected in true multi-infarct dementia where there are only very few (two or three) cortical infarcts. In VaD in general the extent to which the cognitive deficit is patchy is not different from AD, although the domains affected are different.

In VCI subcortical, frontal, and executive pattern of dysfunction is seen in most cases although single lesion VCI, such as after thalamic infarcts, and true multi-infarct VCI, which is uncommon, may have different patterns. Even so, there is commonly a subcortical component to the cognitive impairment, even when the bulk of the cerebrovascular disease does not affect these structures.

That VCI is primarily a subcortical condition means that the screening and simple rating tools used in AD are inappropriate. This applies particularly to the Mini-Mental State Examination (MMSE) which is sensitive to language and memory, involvement of neither of which is predominant in VCI. Instruments that include assessment of frontal, executive, and subcortical function are required. Single tests such as trailmaking, verbal fluency, and digit-symbol substitution can be particularly sensitive and others such as the EXIT25, CLOX, and a modification of the ADAS-Cog termed VaDAS-Cog all represent appropriate steps in this direction. Test batteries that may be able to separate AD and subcortical VCI are now being reported but are not yet widely validated.

Severity of dementia

Current criteria define dementia on the basis of a clear loss of cognitive function, usually sufficient to impair activities of daily living. This is a late stage and, given that the course of cerebrovascular disease is modifiable, will inappropriately deny early cases the best opportunity for secondary preventive measures by failing to detect them.

Leukoaraiosis

The development of CT and MRI scanning led to the identification of periventricular and deep white matter changes which are termed leukoaraiosis [7]. Its cognitive consequences were initially uncertain but more recent work with sensitive tests of cognition has shown that leukoaraiosis is associated with neuropsychological deficits, particularly the attention and speed components of executive function [8–10]. Lesions in the deep gray matter (polioaraiosis) have a greater effect than leukoaraiosis [11]. Longitudinal studies have now also demonstrated a correlation between increasing leukoaraiosis and declining cognition [12,13], implying that treatments to prevent leukoaraiosis progressing might protect cognition.

Lesion volume (or number)

Early work suggested that an infarct volume over 20 cm^3 and in particular of 50 to 100 cm^3 distinguished between VaD and "senile dementia" [14]. However, both dementia and cognitive impairment can exist with much smaller infarct volumes, usually in the range of 1 cm^3 to 30 cm^3, and the correlation between infarct volume and neuropsychological deficit is poor. This is not surprising as site is more important than size and means that there is no precise volume of infarction that can reliably predict VaD other than at meaninglessly large volumes. The current criteria are not, in any case, concerned with infarct volumes but concentrate on numbers of infarcts. While, in subcortical regions, the number of infarcts correlates more closely with cognitive loss than infarct volume, infarcts by themselves are found in less than 50% of cases of established VaD. Microvascular disease, incomplete infarction, and leukoaraiosis are all also crucial in impairing cognition and this further weakens the correlation between infarct volume or number and cognitive status. Infarct volume should not therefore form part of the criteria for VCI.

Lesion site

Lesion site, both for infarcts and other degrees of cerebrovascular damage, is crucial and lesions located at sites such as the thalamus, for example, can be devastating. However, the most important locations are disputed, partly because of the application of variable methods to differing populations, and there is no good way of weighting the cognitive consequences of a lesion according to its location. Magnetic resonance imaging tractography may well lead to the ability to do this but for the present, special emphasis on individual sites is impractical in the formulation of criteria, except perhaps for involvement of the thalamus.

Multiple types and etiologies of vascular dementia

The term "vascular dementia" replaced "multi-infarct dementia" as multiple infarcts are not the only etiology of VCI. All of the current criteria largely treat VaD as a single condition and imply a single etiology and treatment. This is erroneous, since vascular lesions capable of causing cognitive loss arise from many different etiologies and degrees of cerebral damage, and differing causes require different treatments. Each diagnosis of VCI should be accompanied by a statement of etiology as it is this that is most closely linked with secondary preventative therapies.

Atrophy

Atrophy is largely ignored in the current criteria and is often assumed to be due to degenerative dementia; its presence is sometimes used as an argument against a patient having VaD. However, atrophy is a common feature in cerebrovascular disease, even where this is limited to leukoaraiosis, and may progress at the same rate in VaD, AD, and Lewy body dementia [15]. The process can begin without definite vascular events and comprises primarily a relative increase in lateral ventricle volume, suggesting central atrophy. Despite being largely ignored in the current criteria, cognitive impairment correlates better with ventricular enlargement than with infarct volume.

Inclusion of post-stroke dementia

Over one-quarter of patients admitted with stroke become demented but much of this is due to coexistent degenerative dementia, either pre-existent or developed subsequently [16,17]. Most of these cases therefore fall outside pure VaD and might best be considered as mixed dementia unless there is a high level of confidence that only cerebrovascular disease is present.

Mixed dementia

Over the past decade, there has been another major change with the increasing recognition of mixed dementia, where VaD coexists with other causes of dementia, particularly AD. Eighty percent of the elderly have evidence of cerebrovascular disease and mixed VaD and AD may account for up to half of all dementia and may be more common than any other single group [18,19]. Furthermore, the interaction between the vascular component and other components more than doubles the rate of progression when compared to pure AD alone [19,20]. Thus mixed dementia is far more important than was realized when the current criteria were prepared and poses a major problem in that no good method yet exists for identifying mixed dementia in life. Criteria that first select AD-like cases and then subselect those with vascular features might form an excellent basis for doing so; unfortunately this is precisely what the current criteria for VaD do and it is very likely that much of the reported data about VaD are in fact about mixed disease, albeit not yet recognized as such. Mixed cerebrovascular and degenerative dementia is not included within VCI; where there are two pathologies these should both be clearly enumerated and it is perfectly reasonable to diagnose mixed VCI and AD, for example.

A solution: vascular cognitive impairment

The limitations of the old criteria outlined above have led to the acceptance of the new concept of VCI. However, validated criteria for VCI are awaited. Development of these will require alternative rating scales and screening tools that focus on the cognitive domains most affected in vascular disease and a detailed guideline to this and other aspects of the evaluation of VCI has recently been published [21]. The identification of patients with VCI will lead to the identification of risk factors for VCI and in turn will allow the identification of presymptomatic subjects, a stage termed "brain-at-risk" [22] (Figure 4A.1). Vascular

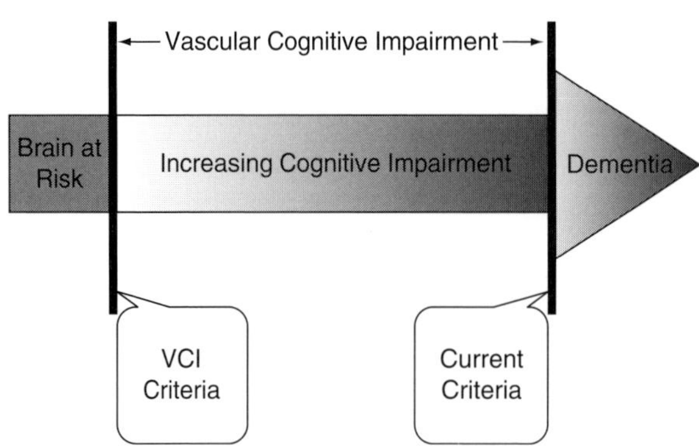

Figure 4A.1 The concept of "brain-at-risk" and vascular cognitive impairment compared to vascular dementia.

cognitive impairment and "brain-at-risk" are the most appropriate stages for early secondary and primary preventative therapy respectively. The lack of formal criteria for VCI in no way prevents clinicians from using the concept now. The key is to identify those patients whose cognition may be impaired, partially or wholly, through cerebrovascular disease. In doing this it is crucial not to dismiss small quantities of infarction and leukoaraiosis etc., as has so often been done in the past. Once identified, risk factor modification is required to reduce the rate of progression. The intent is to prevent dementia from ever developing.

References

1. Hachinski VC, Bowler JV. Vascular dementia. *Neurology* 1993; **43**: 2159–60.
2. World Health Organization. *The ICD-10 Classification of Mental and Behavioural Disorders. Diagnostic Criteria for Research.* Geneva, World Health Organization, 1993.
3. American Psychiatric Association. *Diagnostic and Statistical Manual of Mental Disorders*, 4th edn. Washington, DC, American Psychiatric Association, 1994.
4. Roman GC, Tatemichi TK, Erkinjuntti T, *et al.* Vascular dementia: diagnostic criteria for research studies. Report of the NINDS-AIREN international workshop. *Neurology* 1993; **43**: 250–60.
5. Chui HC, Victoroff JI, Margolin D, *et al.* Criteria for the diagnosis of ischemic vascular dementia proposed by the State of California Alzheimer's Disease Diagnostic and Treatment Centers. *Neurology* 1992; **42** 473–80.
6. Bowler JV Hachinski V. Criteria for vascular dementia: replacing dogma with data. *Arch Neurol* 2000; **57**(2): 170–1.
7. Hachinski VC, Potter P, Merskey H. Leuko-araiosis. *Arch Neurol* 1987; **44**: 21–3.
8. Jokinen H, Kalska H, Mantyla R, *et al.* Cognitive profile of subcortical ischemic vascular disease. *J Neurol Neurosurgery Psychiatry* 2006; **77**(1): 28–33.
9. Prins ND, van Dijk EJ, den Heijer T, *et al.* Cerebral small-vessel disease, and decline in information processing speed, executive function and memory. *Brain* 2005; **128**(9): 2034–41.
10. van der Flier WM, van Straaten ECW, Barkhof F, *et al.* on behalf of the LADIS Study Group. Small vessel disease and general cognitive function in nondisabled elderly: the LADIS study. *Stroke* 2005; **36**(10): 2116–20.
11. Gold G, Kovari E, Herrmann FR, *et al.* Cognitive consequences of thalamic, basal ganglia, and deep white matter lacunes in brain aging and dementia. *Stroke* 2005; **36**(6): 1184–8.
12. Garde E, Lykke Mortensen E, Rostrup E, Paulson OB. Decline in intelligence is associated with progression in white matter hyperintensity volume. *J Neurol Neurosurgery Psychiatry* 2005; **76**(9): 1289–91.
13. Schmidt R, Ropele S, Enzinger C, *et al.* White matter lesion progression, brain atrophy, and cognitive decline: the Austrian stroke prevention study. *Ann Neurol* 2005; **58**(4): 610–16.
14. Tomlinson BE, Blessed G, Roth M. Observations on the brains of demented old people. *J Neurol Sci* 1970; **11**: 205–42.
15. O'Brien JT, Paling S, Barber R, *et al.* Progressive brain atrophy on serial MRI in dementia with Lewy bodies, AD, and vascular dementia. *Neurology* 2001; **56**(10): 1386–8.
16. Barba R, Martínez-Espinosa S, Rodríguez-Garcia E, *et al.* Poststroke dementia: clinical features and risk factors. *Stroke* 2000; **31**(7): 1494–501.

17. Desmond DW, Moroney JT, Paik MC, *et al.* Frequency and clinical determinants of dementia after ischemic stroke. *Neurology* 2000; **54**(5): 1124–31.
18. Neuropathology Group of the Medical Research Council Cognitive Function and Ageing Study (MRC CFAS). Pathological correlates of late-onset dementia in a multicentre, community-based population in England and Wales. *Lancet* 2001; **357**(9251): 169–75.
19. Snowdon DA, Greiner LH, Mortimer JA, *et al.* Brain infarction and the clinical expression of Alzheimer disease. The nun study. *JAMA* 1997; **227**: 813–17.
20. Heyman A, Fillenbaum GG, Welsh-Bohmer KA, *et al.* Cerebral infarcts in patients with autopsy-proven Alzheimer's disease: CERAD, part XVIII. Consortium to Establish a Registry for Alzheimer's Disease. *Neurology* 1998; **51**(1): 159–62.
21. Hachinski V, Iadecola C, Petersen RC, *et al.* National Institute of Neurological Disorders and Stroke–Canadian Stroke Network Vascular Cognitive Impairment Harmonization Standards. *Stroke* 2006; **37**(9): 2220–41.
22. Hachinski VC. Preventable senility: a call for action against the vascular dementias. *Lancet* 1992; **340**: 645–7.

Chapter 4B

Debate: is vascular dementia more common in some parts of the world?

Suvarna Alladi and R. Stewart

Yes

Suvarna Alladi

While the jury is out on geographic differences in prevalence of vascular dementia (VaD), variability clearly exists in the distribution of factors that impact development of VaD. To substantiate this response, evidence will be provided from epidemiological surveys, memory clinic, and neuropathological and cardiovascular risk factor studies that have used standardized and reliable methodology

The definition of VaD has undergone many modifications in the past and several diagnostic criteria exist, but in its most constructive use, the term refers to "dementia due to cerebrovascular disease." While it is very heterogeneous in its causation, clinical course, imaging, and pathology, common factors operating are brain injury caused by vascular disease leading to cognitive impairment.

Criticisms abound regarding the usefulness of the "VaD" construct and reasons often cited include its wide heterogeneity, frequent co-occurrence with Alzheimer's disease (AD) pathology, and etiological significance of "incidental" vascular lesions in patients with dementia. However, there are many more reasons that support its existence as an independent clinical entity. First, there is no doubt that VaD exists as a "pure" entity as confirmed by neuropathological studies and that its frequency in consecutive autopsy series has been found to be quite high [1,2]. Epidemiological studies from both developed and developing countries have also shown that VaD is a common cause of dementia, accounting for 25% to 47% of dementias [3]. Further, unlike AD, VaD is amenable to prevention and treatment and therefore there is a pressing need to study VaD and understand factors that protect or predispose to it

It is now clear that VaD is not a single entity, but represents a complex dementia subtype that occurs as a result of interaction between vascular risk factors, such as hypertension, diabetes,

Dementia: A Global Approach, ed. Ennapadam S. Krishnamoorthy, Martin J. Prince, and Jeffrey L. Cummings. Published by Cambridge University Press.

obesity, dyslipidemia, and brain parenchymal changes, such as macro- and micro-infarcts, hemorrhages, white matter changes, and brain atrophy occurring in an aging brain. An accurate diagnosis requires correlating both clinical features *and* brain imaging. Neuropathological studies have shown that with the aid of imaging, diagnosis of VaD can be made with reasonably good specificity, with existing criteria although sensitivity continues to be low leading to possible underestimation of disease [2].

Developing countries have a rapidly aging population and it is projected that 71% of dementia cases will be in the developing world and hence, absolute numbers of VaD, the second most common type of dementia is likely to be much higher here [3]. Coupled with inadequate healthcare services, VaD is bound to be a bigger problem in developing countries

Risk factors that predispose to VaD are similar to those of cerebrovascular disease. Age, hypertension, especially midlife systolic blood pressure, cardiac disease, peripheral vascular disease, white matter lesions, diabetes mellitus, alcohol consumption, cigarette smoking, hypercholesterolemia, and homocysteinemia are associated with a high risk of stroke and VaD [4–6]. Clear differences are demonstrated in prevalence and incidence of cardiovascular risk factors between high, middle, and low income countries. Cardiovascular disease burden is high in developing countries and has been attributed to the increasing incidence of atherosclerotic diseases, perhaps due to urbanization, epidemiological transition and higher risk factor levels, the relatively early age at which they manifest, the large sizes of the population, and the high proportion of individuals who are young adults or middle-aged in these countries [7]. Higher prevalence of vascular risk factors is likely to increase the burden of VaD in these countries.

Stroke, the overt manifestation of cerebrovascular disease, is one of the most important risk factors for VaD and it is a bigger problem in developing countries than in the developed parts of the world. Strong evidence for ethnic and geographic differences in VaD comes from stroke studies across the world and global estimates of stroke burden indicate a clear difference between countries. Stroke burden is increasing rapidly in developing countries (124% and 107% increases in stroke mortality among men and women in developing countries versus 78% and 56% increases, respectively, in the developed countries). Western studies, on the other hand have demonstrated a reducing incidence of stroke, attributable to improvements in primary prevention of stroke [8]. Since studies have consistently shown that up to 64% of persons who have experienced a stroke have some degree of cognitive impairment [9] with up to a third developing frank dementia [10], the burden of VaD is likely to be much higher in developing countries.

Considerable differences exist in subtypes of stroke among people of different ethnicities. These differences are likely to impact regional patterns and outcome of VaD. Hemorrhagic strokes are more common in Asian countries than in the West, probably due to uncontrolled hypertension [11]. Patterns of vascular mechanisms also differ, and intracranial large and small artery disease predominate in Asia as reflected in both stroke and VaD studies [12,13]. Further, stroke in developing countries affects a younger population.

Table 4B.1 Prevalence of dementia, AD, and VaD in epidemiological studies

Country	All dementia (%)	AD (%)	VaD (%)	Reference
Canada	8	5.1	1.5	CSHA working group [16]
Europe	6.4	4.4	1.6	Lobo *et al.* [17]
China	3.1	2	0.9	Zhang *et al.* [18]
India	3.4	1.6	1.5	Shaji *et al.* [19]
Korea	10.1	5.2	2.1	Jhoo *et al.* [20]

Silent brain infarcts, i.e., infarcts in individuals without clinical manifestation of stroke, are detected in 20% of healthy elderly people and up to 50% of patients in selected series [13,14]. They are associated with subtle deficits in physical and cognitive function that commonly go unnoticed. Moreover, the presence of silent infarcts more than doubles the risk of subsequent stroke and dementia [15]. In view of the variability in cardiovascular risk factors, stroke patterns, and life expectancy, the role of silent brain infarcts in influencing VaD patterns needs to be explored.

A wide variability in worldwide prevalence of VaD has been reported by most epidemiological studies. Reasons cited include methodological differences in diagnosis and sociocultural factors in attitudes towards dementia. A true ethnic variability due to lifestyle and genetic factors does remain a possibility. Variations in VaD prevalence have however been demonstrated across countries (Table 4B.1), and across different regions in the same country [18]. Inter-ethnic differences in age-standardized dementia prevalence were demonstrated in Singapore. Malays had twice the risk for AD as Chinese, and Indians had more than twice the risk for AD and VaD than Chinese [21]. Prevalence of VaD in Japan has also shown changes over time with demographic shifts in the country's population [22].

Prevalence of a disease is a reflection both on its incidence as well as outcome, and has not been adequately investigated in developing countries. Conclusions on geographic differences in VaD should take into account incidence data as well as duration of disease in different populations.

Accurate diagnosis of VaD requires correlation of clinical features with imaging by a trained clinician. This approach to diagnosis is feasible in memory clinics, where dementia patients are systematically evaluated for cause and subtype. Useful information can be obtained by comparing frequency of VaD in memory clinic populations across the world. Vascular dementia was diagnosed in 5.6% to 8.7% of patients in developed countries, which is considerably less than the prevalence of about 26.2% in developing country studies [23,24].

The frequent coexistence of AD and VaD (mixed dementia) further complicates the issue of determining differences in dementia subtype prevalence across the world since VaD criteria do not reliably differentiate mixed dementia and pure VaD [2]. Current thoughts point towards using the umbrella term "vascular cognitive impairment" (VCI) to include pure VaD, mixed dementia, and milder forms of vascular cognitive impairment since they represent a spectrum of cognitive disorders caused by cerebrovascular disease [25]. Mixed dementia appears to play a bigger role in late-onset dementia as opposed to early-onset dementia (31.4% vs. 5.9%). Differences in life expectancy that exist between countries are therefore likely to impact the proportion of AD, pure VaD, and mixed dementia in these populations. Significantly, evidence for age-related increase in VaD prevalence is weaker when compared to the exponential increase in AD prevalence [18]. Studying mixed dementia will thereby enhance understanding of impact of age on differences in dementia due to cerebrovascular disease. Comparative studies of age-normalized populations will generate a clearer pattern of VaD, AD, and mixed dementia across different age groups within specific ethnic communities.

In an attempt to harmonize research methodology in this area with the aim to identify and accurately diagnose VCI, particularly in the early stages, The National Institute for Neurological Disorders and Stroke (NINDS) and the Canadian Stroke Network have developed common standards in clinical diagnosis, epidemiology, brain imaging, neuropathology, experimental models, genetics, and clinical trials to recommend minimum, common, clinical, and research standards for the description and study of vascular cognitive impairment [26]. Efforts are underway to put these recommendations into practice and a clearer pattern of VCI in different areas is likely to emerge.

The pertinent questions should therefore center more on elucidating differences in burden of VaD, its risk factors, subtypes, and outcome in different countries and ethnic populations. Variability exists in the above factors between places, and a greater understanding of this variability in future research is necessary, in order to reduce the global burden of cognitive impairment due to cerebrovascular disease.

No

R. Stewart

For those who do not wish to read any further, my answer is not strictly "No," but really just that the question is at best unhelpful and at worst dangerously misleading. The reason is that "vascular dementia (VaD)" is an entity which is untenable and outdated and which should be shed as soon as possible – by epidemiology at least, if not by all dementia research. To continue to discuss "VaD" as if we know what we are talking about is no longer an exercise of academic navel gazing (if it ever was) but now has real potential negative consequences.

First, some history. Once upon a time, around the middle of the twentieth century, most late-onset dementia was assumed to be vascular in origin. Seminal postmortem research in the late 1960s and early 1970s demonstrated that Alzheimer's disease (AD), previously thought to be principally a pre-senile dementia, was in fact also likely to underlie the majority of late-onset cases. However, many cases had evidence of clearly significant cerebrovascular disease, measured in those days by volume of infarction. This led to what at the time was an entirely appropriate division of most dementia into AD and multi-infarct dementia. Multi-infarct dementia was later renamed "vascular dementia," in recognition of the observation that vascular pathology underlying dementia was not confined to multiple infarctions. A "mixed dementia" category was originally acknowledged but received little or no subsequent research. However, it is becoming increasingly apparent that most dementia has mixed causation and a distinction between AD and VaD as diagnoses is no longer tenable.

Many things have changed since the 1960s and there is no reason why diagnoses should not also evolve. People dying with dementia in Western nations 40 years ago would have been likely to have much more florid cerebrovascular pathology than would be expected now because there were few interventions to prevent or control the most important vascular risk factors. They would also have been much more likely to have discrete rather than mixed pathology simply because they were dying at younger ages. It is a matter of simple common sense that people with dementia in their ninth and tenth decades are highly likely to have mixed underlying pathology and yet a diagnostic system persists which assumes that clinical cases can be divided into mutually exclusive categories. Another important change over the last 40 years is that much more sophisticated techniques are routinely available in many clinical settings for evaluating subclinical vascular disease. Early assessment tools such as the Hachinski Ischemic Scale [27] focused on ascertaining by history and examination whether there was evidence of cerebral infarction, whereas clinical diagnostic decisions in many settings now have to take into account CT and/or MRI findings which may identify much more subtle vascular changes. These changes may be contributory but are unlikely to represent sole causes of cognitive decline, since they are present in many older people who show no signs of dementia.

The fundamental problem with dementia subclassification in clinical and epidemiological research is that it is an exercise in "guess the pathology." This may be easy enough when someone aged 60 presents with dementia following a series of strokes, in whom co-occurring AD is statistically very unlikely. However, for cases of dementia in their 80s and 90s, this guesswork is simply not appropriate, for VaD at least. The reason it is used at all has probably arisen from AD research. If a person with late-onset dementia has no potential cause identified (i.e., principally has no evidence of significant cerebrovascular disease or a medical condition known to cause dementia such as Parkinson's disease) then it is reasonable to assume that significant Alzheimer pathology is present and, from what we understand so far, probably AD is the principal cause. The same process cannot be carried out for VaD because Alzheimer pathology cannot (yet) be identified and excluded in life and in most cases it is simply not appropriate to assume that, just because there is evidence of vascular disease, this is the sole underlying cause of dementia (since many people with significant vascular disease do not have dementia). The only way this can be attempted is by ascertaining the temporal relationship between known or suspected infarction episodes and the previous course of cognitive decline. This relies heavily on an adequate informant account and is very difficult to carry out with any respectable degree of reliability: something which has been demonstrated in a research context but which really should be obvious to anyone who has had any clinical experience in dementia diagnosis.

Given these issues, it is not at all surprising that research diagnostic criteria for VaD have performed poorly when evaluated – poor agreement between different diagnostic instruments [28], poor inter-rater reliability for most instruments [28,29], and poor agreement with pathological findings [1,30,31]. It is also not surprising that the most problematic aspects of the "diagnosis" involve the attempts to define likely causation through inquiring about the previous course of cognitive decline or the pattern of cognitive deficits [32,33]. The Hachinski Ischemic Scale, which principally aims to identify the presence of significant cerebrovascular disease, was found to have the best performance in terms of inter-rater agreement [28]. However, this instrument was never intended to be a diagnostic assessment and its developer has been one of the strongest critics of "VaD" as a construct [34].

If diagnostic schedules for VaD cannot be demonstrated to be reliable when specifically evaluated in single centers, then it is doubtful whether anything can be inferred from variation in international prevalence rates. Even if criteria could be reliably applied, at best such a comparison of prevalence rates might give an idea of variation in comorbidity between cerebrovascular disease and dementia. This will be determined by a large number of factors, influencing both chance co-occurrence (the age structure of the population, the underlying risk of cerebrovascular disease, and the underlying risk of dementia) as well as reasons why the two may occur together more commonly than expected. It is not at all clear whether there is any benefit to science or public health to be gained by describing the frequency of a construct which attempts to encompass all these processes, and which researchers cannot even agree how to define.

The continued use of "VaD" as a research category not only perpetuates a myth that it can be adequately defined, but also may have genuine adverse consequences. One feature of recent clinical trials in VaD has been the difficulties encountered in recruiting sufficient numbers of people who fulfill clinical criteria. From the author's impression of some of the resulting presentations, it does not look likely that the prospect of trials of future agents in this group would be greeted with enthusiasm. "Vascular dementia" already receives very little research as an outcome compared to "AD," partly because as a diagnosis it falls between traditional clinical specialties but also probably because of the problems encountered with its definition. Even "dementia" itself is problematic in relation to vascular risk factors because standard criteria focus particularly on memory deficits with AD in mind [35], and because the decision about whether cognitive decline is causing global functional impairment may be difficult or impossible when another equally disabling condition, such as stroke, is present. "Vascular cognitive impairment" has been proposed as an alternative construct [36] although with no diagnostic criteria and therefore not something which can be applied yet in prevalence studies. However, VaD continues to be cited widely as a diagnosis and the problems with this are not yet adequately recognised beyond its research field. This potentially leads to the following:

1. The more the VaD "diagnosis" is quoted in research outputs, the more it is perceived to have external validity and something which can be incorporated into clinical decision-making and policy.
2. If VaD is recognized as problematic by the research community and yet there is still an expectation to subcategorize dementia, "VaD," however defined, is most likely to be treated as an exclusion criterion. Therefore, any group of people defined by this "diagnosis" will suffer from a limited evidence base for interventions.
3. If, as seems to be a growing trend, the absence of an evidence-based intervention means, in reality, no intervention at all, then people with a VaD diagnosis may be profoundly disadvantaged.

The argument presented here is that "VaD" is a category which should no longer be used in research because it cannot be applied with adequate reliability (i.e., consistency between research groups) or validity (i.e., defining underlying pathological processes). It is further argued that its continued use as a "diagnosis" both in research and clinical practice is not evidence-based and is probably counterproductive. This is not to say that "VaD" as a field of research is problematic; indeed, an enormous amount of progress has been made over the past ten years in advancing understanding of how risk factors for cardiovascular disease also increase risk of dementia. A key finding, however, is that the resulting dementia syndrome is not confined to the traditional "multi-infarct" picture but encompasses AD as well. Cerebrovascular pathology is therefore much better conceptualized as a causal pathway to a wide range of dementia syndromes, rather than as a means to define particular subgroups – apart from in relatively rare instances, such as strategic infarct dementias or early-onset multi-infarct syndromes.

International variation in dementia risk is an important issue, and vascular factors are likely to play an important part in this simply because they are probably the most important environmental risk factors for dementia and because there are well-recognized (and substantial) international differences in risk profiles. However the question posed for this debate is wholly inadequate for addressing this issue. The question which *should* be posed is twofold: (1) How much international heterogeneity is there in dementia risk? (2) To what extent can this heterogeneity be accounted for by national differences in vascular risk profile? These questions are extremely pressing ones for public health and policy because of the huge economic importance of dementia prevalence and rapid changes in both age structures and cardiovascular disease prevalence in many nations. However, the answers are unlikely to be easily achieved and may rest on study designs from which it is very difficult to draw firm conclusions. The most obvious of these is a concerted attempt to describe and compare dementia prevalence reliably across a large number of nations and/or within-nation subpopulations (e.g., migrant groups). Early evidence can be said to be in place through the two-site Ibadan–Indianapolis project where both prevalence and incidence of dementia were found to be substantially lower in a Nigerian compared to a Black American population [37,38], the former also having substantially lower cardiovascular risk. However, confounding is always a major problem in ecological study designs (i.e., the two populations are different in many other respects) and may be problematic even in multisite designs such as that of the 10/66 Research Program [39]. A second, more ambitious approach would be through a time series study where repeated surveys are carried out to investigate changes in age-specific prevalence of dementia in a population whose vascular risk status has also been changing. Again, there is the problem of confounding and the difficulty in inferring causality.

In conclusion, the role of vascular factors in determining national prevalence of dementia is an important public health issue. However, it may only be possible to address this question through relatively weak research designs (in terms of ability to infer causality), since stronger ones (such as randomized controlled trials) are unlikely to be feasible. What is much more certain is that a comparison of "VaD" prevalence rates is both fundamentally flawed and positively unhelpful.

References

1. Gold G, Giannakopoulos P, Montes-Paixao Júnior C, *et al.* Sensitivity and specificity of newly proposed clinical criteria for possible vascular dementia. *Neurology* 1997; **49**: 690–4
2. Knopman DS, Parisi JE, Boeve BF, *et al.* Vascular dementia in a population-based autopsy study. *Arch Neurol* 2003; **60**: 569–75.
3. Kalaria RN, Maestre GE, Arizaga R, *et al.* Alzheimer's disease and vascular dementia in developing countries: prevalence, management, and risk factors. *Lancet Neurol* 2008; **7**: 812–26.
4. Skoog I, Lernfelt B, Landahl S, *et al.* 15 year longitudinal study of blood pressure and dementia. *Lancet Neurol* 1996; **347**: 1141–5.
5. Boston PF, Dennis MS, Jagger C. Factors associated with vascular dementia in an elderly community population. *Int J Geriatr Psychiatry* 1999; **14**: 761–6.
6. Ross GW, Pertrivitch H, White LR, *et al.* Characterization of risk factors for vascular dementia: the Honolulu-Asia Aging Study. *Neurology* 1999; **53**: 337–43.
7. Yusuf S, Reddy S, Ounpuu S, Anand S. Global burden of cardiovascular diseases: Part I: general considerations, the epidemiological transition, risk factors, and impact of urbanization. *Circulation* 2001; **104**: 2746–53.
8. Paul SL, Srikanth VK, Thrift AG. The large and growing burden of stroke. *Curr Drug Targets* 2007; **8**: 786–93.
9. Pohjasvaara T, Erkinjuntti T, Vataja R, Kaste M. Dementia three months after stroke: baseline frequency and effect of different definitions of dementia in the Helsinki Stroke Aging Memory Study (SAM) cohort. *Stroke* 1997; **28**: 785–92.
10. Tatemichi TK, Desmond DW, Stern Y, *et al.* Prevalence of dementia after stroke depends on diagnostic criteria. *Neurology* 1992; **42**: 413.
11. Das SK, Banerjee TK. Stroke: Indian Scenario. *Circulation* 2008; **118**: 2719–24.
12. Alladi S, Kaul S, Meena AK, *et al.* Pattern of vascular dementia in India: study of clinical features, imaging, and vascular mechanisms from a hospital dementia registry. *J Stroke Cerebrovasc Dis* 2006; **15**: 49–56.
13. Alluri RV, Mohan V, Komandur S, *et al.* MTHFR C677T gene mutation as a risk factor for arterial stroke: a hospital based study. *Eur J Neurol* 2005; **12**: 40–4.

13. Leary MC, Saver JF. Annual incidence of first silent stroke in the United States: a preliminary estimate. *Cerebrovasc Dis* 2003; **16**: 280–5.

14. Vermeer SE, Longstreth WT. Jr, Koudstaal PJ. Silent brain infarcts: a systematic review. *Lancet Neurol* 2007; **6**: 611–19.

15. Vermeer SE, Prins ND, den Heijer T, *et al.* Silent brain infarcts and the risk of dementia and cognitive decline. *N Engl J Med* 2003; **348**: 1215–22.

16. Canadian study of health and aging working group. Canadian study of health and aging: study methods and prevalence of dementia. *CMAJ* 1994; **150**: 899–913.

17. Lobo A, Launer LJ, Fratiglioni L. Prevalence of dementia and major subtypes in Europe: a collaborative study of population-based cohorts. Neurologic Diseases in the Elderly Research Group. *Neurology* 2000; **54**: S4–9.

18. Zhang Z, Zahner GEP, Roman GC, *et al.* Dementia subtypes in China. *Arch Neurol* 2005; **5**: 447–453.

19. Shaji S, Bose S, Verghese A. Prevalence of dementia in an urban population in Kerala, India. *Br J Psychiatry* 2005; **186**: 136–40.

20. Jhoo JH, Kim KW, Huh Y, *et al.* Prevalence of dementia and its subtypes in an elderly urban korean population: results from the Korean Longitudinal Study on Health And Aging (KLoSHA). *Dement Geriatr Cogn Disord* 2008; **26**: 270–6.

21. Sahadevan S, Saw SM, Gao W, *et al.* Ethnic differences in Singapore's dementia prevalence: the stroke, Parkinson's disease, epilepsy, and dementia in Singapore study. *J Am Geriatr Soc* 2008; **56**: 2061–8.

22. Kiyohara Y, Yoshitake T, Kato I, *et al.* Changing patterns in the prevalence of dementia in a Japanese community: the Hisayama study. *Gerontology* 1994; **40**: 29–35.

23. Sheng B, Law CB, Yeung KM. Characteristics and diagnostic profile of patients seeking dementia care in a memory clinic in Hong Kong. *Int Psychogeriatr* 2008; **23**: 1–9.

24. Shelley BP, Al Khabouri J. The spectrum of dementia: frequency, causes and clinical profile. A national referral hospital-based study in Oman. *Dement Geriatr Cogn Disord* 2007; **24**: 280–7.

25. Bowler JV, Hachinski V. The concept of vascular cognitive impairment. In: Erkinjuntti T, Gauthier S, eds. *Vascular Cognitive Impairment.* London, Martin Dunitz. 2002; 9–25.

26. Hachinski V, Iadecola C, Petersen RC, *et al.* National Institute of Neurological Disorders and Stroke–Canadian Stroke Network Vascular Cognitive Impairment Harmonization Standards. *Stroke* 2006; **37**: 2220–41.

27. Hachinski VC, Iliff LD, Zilhka E, *et al.* Cerebral blood flow in dementia. *Arch Neurol* 1975; **32**: 632–7.

28. Chui HC, Mack W, Jackson JE, *et al.* Clinical criteria for the diagnosis of vascular dementia. *Arch Neurol* 2000; **57**: 191–6.

29. Lopez OL, Larumbe MR, Becker JT, *et al.* Reliability of NINDS-AIREN clinical criteria for the diagnosis of vascular dementia. *Neurology* 1994; **44**: 1240–5.

30. Holmes C, Cairns N, Lantos P, *et al.* Validity of current clinical criteria for Alzheimer's disease, vascular dementia and dementia with Lewy bodies. *Br J Psychiatry* 1999; **174**: 45–50.

31. Gold G, Bouras C, Canuto A, *et al.* Clinicopathological validation study of four sets of clinical criteria for vascular dementia. *Am J Psychiatry* 2002; **159**: 82–7.

32. Fischer P, Gatterer G, Marterer A, *et al.* Course characteristics in the differentiation of dementia of the Alzheimer type and multi-infarct dementia. *Acta Psychiatr Scand* 1990; **81**: 551–3.

33. Boston PF, Dennis MS, Jagger C, *et al.* Unequal distribution of cognitive deficits in vascular dementia – is this a valid criterion in the ICD-10? *Int J Geriatr Psychiatry* 2001; **16**: 422–6.

34. Bowler JV, Hachinski V. Criteria for vascular dementia: replacing dogma with data. *Arch Neurol* 2000; **57**: 170–1.

35. American Psychiatric Association. *Diagnostic and Statistical Manual of Mental Disorders, Fourth Edition*. Washington, DC, APA, 1994.

36. O'Brien JT, Erkinjuntti T, Reisberg B, *et al.* Vascular cognitive impairment. *Lancet Neurol* 2003; **2**: 89–98.

37. Hendrie HC, Osuntokun BO, Hall KS, *et al.* Prevalence of Alzheimer's disease and dementia in two communities: Nigerian Africans and African Americans. *Am J Psychiatry* 1995; **152**: 1485–92.

38. Hendrie HC, Ogunniyi A, Hall KS, *et al.* Incidence of dementia and Alzheimer disease in 2 communities. *JAMA* 2001; **285**: 739–47.

39. Prince M, Ferri CP, Acosta D, *et al.* The protocols for the 10/66 Dementia Research Group population-based research programme. *BMC Public Health* 2007; **7**: 165.

Cross-cultural issues of global significance

Infections and dementia: the view from a developing nation

P. Satishchandra and Vijayan Joy

Medicine is a science of uncertainty and an art of probability.
William Osler

Introduction

The importance of dementia in a country like India can be inferred when one considers that by the year 2030, about 70% of the patients with cognitive and behavioral decline will be living in developing nations. One needs to consider a number of etiological possibilities while dealing with a patient presenting with dementia. The most common causes are degenerative, vascular, or mixed. However, in countries such as India, infections and nutritional deficiencies have to be entertained in the list of differentials. Even though they form a small group when dementia is considered as a whole, they assume significance due to the widespread prevalence of tuberculosis and cysticercosis. Adding fuel to this fire is the emergence of HIV as an epidemic in India. Human immunodeficiency virus is associated with considerable social stigmatization, which, together with the numerous and complex psychosocial issues, brings a certain complexity to the care of the patient with AIDS dementia complex.

There are a few published studies from India, looking at the prevalence of infection-associated dementia. In a prospective hospital-based study from Bangalore, it was found that infection was the third most common cause [1]. Another study from Lucknow, on 124 patients, showed that 10 were secondary to tuberculosis and 10 due to cysticercosis [2].

There are a number of infections where cognitive decline can be the presenting feature. Some of the causes are enumerated in Table 5A.1.

In addition, there are conditions wherein cognitive and behavioral impairments form important sequelae to a monophasic infective process. This is seen secondary to a wide variety of infections including Herpes simplex encephalitis, cerebral malaria, and Japanese B encephalitis. The subsections that follow will

Dementia: A Global Approach, ed. Ennapadam S. Krishnamoorthy, Martin J. Prince, and Jeffrey L. Cummings. Published by Cambridge University Press.

Table 5A.1 Dementia associated with conventional and unconventional agents

Dementia associated with conventional agents	
Viral	**Fungal**
HIV-associated dementia	Cryptococcal
Subacute sclerosing panencephalitis (SSPE)	Candida
Progressive multifocal leukoencephalopathy (PML)	Aspergillosis
Bacterial/Mycobacterial	**Parasitic**
Tuberculous infection	Neurocysticercosis
Whipple's disease	Toxoplasmosis
Brucellosis	
Spirochetal	
Neurosyphilis	
Lyme disease	
Dementia associated with unconventional agents	
Creutzfeldt–Jacob disease	Kuru
Gerstmann–Straussler–Scheinker disease	Fatal familial insomnia

discuss briefly the most commonly occurring infection-related dementias.

HIV-associated dementia/AIDS dementia complex

As per the UNAIDS report [3], there are about six million people living with AIDS in India as of early 2006. Reports from the West suggest that the prevalence of HIV-associated dementia can be as high as 20–25%. However, literature from India has reported a prevalence of only about 2–4% [4,5]. This has been attributed to shorter survival periods, with many of the patients succumbing early to opportunistic infections. Other factors to be considered are absence of any standardized cognitive assessment scale in a multi-linguistic society; differences in the HIV strain, with subtype C being more common in India; and the absence of C-Tat protein. [6]. In contrast to these earlier findings, there has been a recent cross-sectional study reporting a higher prevalence of neurocognitive deficits in asymptomatic seropositive patients from Pune [7].

As a clinician, it is essential to look for possible neuropsychological profiles that would help in identifying the type of dementia one is dealing with. This can be very helpful, as in the case with the primary degenerative dementias. There are a number of studies that have looked at the neuropsychological aspects of AIDS dementia complex. Many of them point towards early involvement of the frontal network system.

In a study carried out on 119 patients with clade C HIV-1, it was found that about 60% of the patients had impairment of fluency, attention, learning, and memory, suggestive of frontal and temporal lobe involvement [8]. Many of these patients had difficulty with complex mental tasks, alternating sequence tests, set-shifting, etc. A positive correlation was also seen between the degree of visuospatial impairment and the immune status. These findings have been replicated in other studies [2,9,10]. One study showed a direct correlation between impairment of executive functioning and advancing age. In addition, these patients were reported to have behavioral symptoms such as apathy, emotional blunting, decreased libido, and excessive tiredness.

Another important aspect of AIDS dementia complex is the presence of motor symptoms and signs. This can thus be considered as a form of subcortical dementia. Many of these patients exhibit mild parkinsonian features, with slowness of activity, gait instability, tremulousness, etc. There are a number of classificatory systems for AIDS dementia complex, including the one put forward by the American Academy of Neurology [11], that take into account these various manifestations.

Before labeling a patient as having AIDS dementia complex, one has to rule out opportunistic infections. This aspect has been highlighted in the study carried out by Deshpande *et al.*, wherein only 22% of patients out of a total of 300 HIV-seropositive patients had central nervous system (CNS) involvement not directly related to an underlying opportunistic infection [12].

Patients with HIV-associated dementia should be put on antiretroviral therapy (HAART) as per standard recommendations [13]. In addition, there are recent studies which show beneficial effects of memantine, peptide T inhibitors, serotonin reuptake inhibitors, and 3-hydroxy-3-methylglutaryl-coenzyme A (HMG-CoA) reductase inhibitors. Being beneficial in AIDS, the latter two act by reducing HIV RNA levels in the cerebro spinal fluid (CSF) [14,15].

Neurological opportunistic complications of HIV infection

Infection of the CNS by opportunistic organisms (OIs) is an important aspect in HIV-seropositive patients, with many patients succumbing to these complications even before the development of illness manifestations that can be attributed to the virus per se [16]. The opportunistic complications include infections secondary to *Cryptococcus neoformans, neurotuberculosis, Toxoplasma gondii, JC virus, Cytomegalovirus*, etc.

Clinical presentations of these complications are similar to their usual presentations in a normal host, but in some of the patients they can be milder or at times more aggressive. One also needs to be aware of the possibility of persisting neurocognitive deficits, in spite of successfully treating these opportunistic complications [17].

Most of these opportunistic infections tend to cause dementia by various pathogenetic mechanisms which include meningitis, encephalitis, arteritis, or by obstructing the CSF pathway. They may also present as granulomas, giving rise to focal neurological signs.

Neuroimaging studies, CSF analysis, and serological studies may help in differentiating the various etiologies. In case of cryptococcal infection, imaging studies may show the presence of cortical atrophy, punctuate non-enhancing foci of CSF density correlating with the presence of cryptococci in the Virchow-Robin space or focal lesions consistent with cryptococcomas. Cerebrospinal fluid studies may not show a robust inflammatory response and culture for cryptococci may not be positive [18]. Imaging studies in toxoplasmosis may show multiple ring-enhancing lesions, with predilection for the basal ganglia. Polymerase chain reaction for toxoplasmosis in the CSF is positive in approximately 60% of patients.

Progressive multifocal leukoencephalopathy (PML) presents with cognitive deficits or pyramidal signs. There are reports of it being less common in infections associated with "clade C" HIV virus from India [19]. Imaging studies of the brain with high-resolution MRI can be extremely useful in diagnosing this entity, with non-enhancing multiple white matter changes being seen predominantly involving the parieto-occipital and frontal regions. There are no specific treatment options available. However, HAART definitely has a role to play when PML is associated with HIV infecton.

Neurosyphilis

Neurosyphilis is one of the most commonly associated infections seen in patients with AIDS in the West ranging from 3% to as high as 22% [20,21]. With the advent of multiple broad-spectrum antibiotics its occurrence in isolation, and as one of the reasons for reversible dementia, is almost nil from studies done in the West. However, it continues to be an important cause of dementia, even in the absence of HIV infection, in India. No specific neuropsychological profile was described in these patients, both neurocognitive decline and neurobehavioral disorder being described as occurring independently or in combination. In addition, pupillary abnormalities and other focal neurological signs were described in these individuals. Neuroimaging studies (Figure 5A.1) can also be very heterogeneous, with frequent descriptions of mesial temporal lobe involvement on MR studies. Diagnosis is based on CSF pleocytosis, VDRL (venereal disease research laboratory) test, and confirmatory FTA-ABS (fluorescent treponemal antibody absorption) test. The mainstay of treatment continues to be intravenous crystalline penicillin G, which is to be given at a dose of 2–4 million units every 4 hours for a total of 14–21 days. Further monitoring is by repeating the blood VDRL once every three months for the first year, and thereafter at six-monthly intervals during the second year with the CSF study being repeated at the end of one/two years.

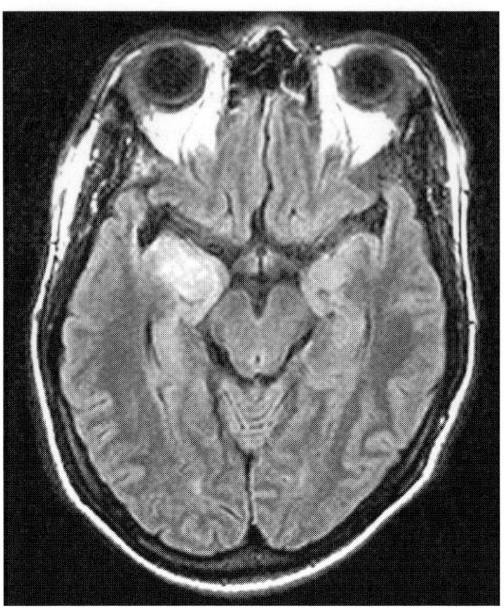

Figure 5A.1 Neurosyphilis: T2W image of the brain which shows hyperintensity of both the mesial temporal regions, left more than right, in a patient presenting with a progressive amnestic syndrome.

CNS tuberculosis

Tuberculosis is one of the highly prevalent infections seen in the Indian subcontinent. It tends to involve multiple organs within the body, the CNS being among the commonest. Involvement of the CNS can be in the form of meningitis, meningoencephalitis, arteritis, venous thrombosis, multiple granulomas, or craniospinal arachnoiditis [22]. It can also cause obstruction to the CSF outflow leading to cognitive decline and hydrocephalus. The meningitis, which is typically basal, can cause arteritis particularly of the perforators supplying the deep gray matter, leading to infarction of the thalamus, basal ganglia, basal forebrain, etc. This can lead to dementia akin to strategically placed infarcts, well described in the vascular dementia literature (see Chapter 4A for more on the pathogenesis of vascular dementia). Neurotuberculosis has achieved greater importance in recent years because of the increase in prevalence of comorbid HIV infection.

The diagnosis is clinched through a combination of screening investigations to rule out other system involvement, neuroimaging, and CSF studies. A high index of clinical suspicion is extremely important, as laboratory investigations may be of only moderate help. Staining for acid-fast bacilli in CSF is positive in only 20–25% of patients, and cultures are positive in 15–20% of patients. Polymerase chain reaction and BACTEC are quicker and more promising. Cerebrospinal fluid adenosine deaminase may also be helpful.

A treatment protocol has been developed jointly by the American Thoracic Society, the Centers for Disease Control and the Infectious Disease Society of North America [23]. The authors recommend 12 months of antituberculous medication, the initial 2 months being isoniazid, rifampicin, pyrazinamide, and ethambutol/streptomycin, followed by 10 months of isoniazid and rifampicin. Early diagnosis and treatment definitely is useful in reversing cognitive deficits associated with neurotuberculosis.

Neurocysticercosis

This is the most common parasitic infection of the brain seen in India and continues to be the most common medical cause of acute or remote symptomatic seizures. Other modes of presentation are headache, either due to multiple cysticercal granulomas (Figure 5A.2) or as a result of obstruction to the CSF outflow by the cystic lesion. Dementia is also one of the recognized presentations of neurocysticercosis. In a study from India, involving 62 patients

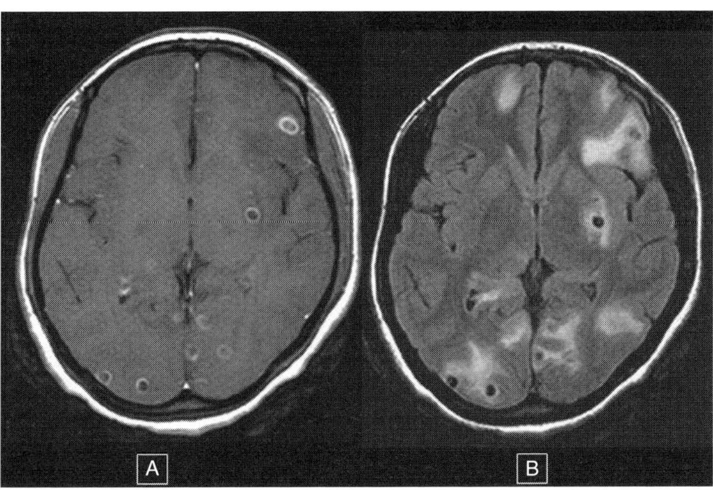

Figure 5A.2 (A and B) Patient with multiple neurocysticercosis: MRI T1W images show multiple cystic lesions with central scolex.

followed over a period of five years, 6% of patients had dementia [24,25,26]. In another study carried out in Mexico, 14 of 90 patients were diagnosed to have dementia as per Diagnostic and Statistical Manual of Mental Disorders, fourth edition (DSM-IV) criteria [27]. Neurocysticercosis can also present with psychiatric manifestations [28]. The treatment of choice is albendazole at a dose of 15 mg/kg body weight for 2–4 weeks. Patients should usually be primed with a short course of steroids to prevent the development of fatal cerebral edema. Dementia of neurocysticercosis is usually reversible, as demonstrated by the Mexican study, wherein almost 80% of the treated patients no longer fulfilled the DSM-IV criteria.

Creutzfeldt–Jacob disease

There are a number of studies from India that have shown the growing prevalence of Creutzfeldt–Jacob disease [29,30]. The importance of Creutzfeldt–Jacob disease had grown in significance following the Colchester hypothesis, which had suggested the root cause of the bovine spongiform encephalopathy was the contamination of animal feeds with human remains from the Ganges [31], a proposal that has been strongly refuted by Indian scientists [32].

The presentation one commonly associates with Creutzfeldt–Jacob disease is one of a rapidly progressive dementia with myoclonus. There are, however, several other variants wherein the presentation could be with progressive cortical blindness, extrapyramidal features, or cerebellar ataxia. Diagnosis is based on EEG which shows periodic triphasic or biphasic sharp wave/spike complexes of 0.5–2.0 Hz on a slow background and MRI changes (Figure 5A.3). The treatment of this disease does however remain a challenge, fatal outcomes being the norm.

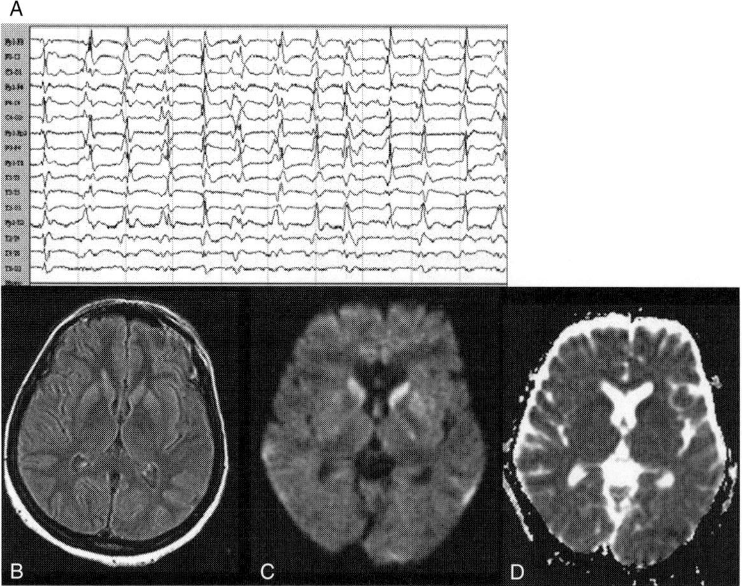

Figure 5A.3 Creutzfeldt–Jacob disease. (A) EEG showing periodic triphasic complexes, occurring at 1 second intervals. (B) T2W FLAIR imaging of the brain showing hyperintensity on the caudate and lentiform nuclei and thalamus. (C) Diffusion-weighted imaging showing signal changes in the caudate and lentiform nuclei and thalamus. (D) Apparent diffusion coefficient: showing restricted diffusion of the above mentioned areas.

Conclusion

Infection continues to be one of the important causes of dementia especially in developing countries. With the upsurge in HIV infection in the last two decades, AIDS dementia has become significant even in the developed world. Further, infections are an important cause of reversible dementia and the astute clinician needs to consider this differential diagnosis especially when confronted with rapidly progressive dementia syndromes, which occur too among younger people.

References

1. Srikanth S, Nagaraj AV. A prospective study of reversible dementias: frequency, causes, clinical profile and results of treatment. *Neurol India* 2005; **53**: 291–4.
2. Jha S, Patel R. Some observations on the spectrum of dementia. *Neurol India* 2004; **52**: 213–14.
3. UNAIDS. *Report on the Global AIDS Epidemic.* Geneva, UNAIDS, 2006.
4. Satishchandra P, Nalini A, Gourie-Devi M, Jayakumar PN, Shankar SK. Profile of neurological disorders associated with HIV/AIDS from South India. *Indian J Med Res* 2000; **111**: 14–23.
5. Sinha S, Satishchandra P. Nervous system involvement in asymptomatic HIV seropositive individuals: a cognitive and electrophysiological study. *Neurol India* 2003; **51**: 466–9.
6. Ranga U, Shankarappa R, Satishchandra P, *et al.* Tat protein of human immunodeficiency virus type 1 subtype C strains is a defective chemokine. *J Virol* 2004; **78**: 2586–90.
7. Riedel D, Ghate M, Nene M, *et al.* Screening for human immunodeficiency virus (HIV) dementia in an HIV clade C-infected population in India. *J Neurovirol* 2006; **12**: 34–8.
8. Gupta JD, Satishchandra P, Gopukumar K, *et al.* Neuropsychological deficits in human immunodeficiency virus type 1 clade C-seropositive adults from South India. *J Neurovirol* 2007; **13**: 195–202.
9. Cysique LA, Maruff P, Brew BJ. The neuropsychological profile of symptomatic AIDS and ADC patients in the pre-HAART era: a meta-analysis. *J Int Neuropsychol Soc* 2006; **12**: 368–82.
10. Sacktor N, Skolasky R, Selnes OA, *et al.* Neuropsychological test profile differences between young and old human immunodeficiency virus-positive individuals. *J Neurovirol* 2007; **13**: 203–9.
11. American Academy of Neurology AIDS Task Force Working Group. Report of a Working Group of the American Academy of Neurology AIDS Task Force. Nomenclature and research case definitions for neurologic manifestations of human immunodeficiency virus-type-1. *Neurology* 1991; **41**: 778–85.
12. Deshpande AK, Patnaik MM. Nonopportunistic neurologic manifestations of the human immunodeficiency virus: an Indian study. *MedGenMed* 2005; **4**(7): 2.
13. Letendre S, Ances B, Gibson S, Ellis RJ. Neurologic complications of HIV disease and their treatment. *Top HIV Med* 2007; **15**: 32–9.
14. Schifitto G, Navia BA, Yiannoutsos CT, *et al.* Memantine and HIV associated cognitive impairment: a neuropsychological and proton magnetic resonance spectroscopy study. *AIDS* 2007; **21**: 1877–86.
15. Heseltine PN, Goodkin K, Atkinson JH, *et al.* Randomized double-blind placebo-controlled trial of peptide T for HIV-associated cognitive impairment. *Arch Neurol* 1998; **55**: 41–51.

16. Santosh V, Shankar SK, Das S, *et al.* Pathological lesions in HIV positive patients. *Indian J Med Res* 1995; **101**: 134–41.

17. Mahadevan A, Shankar SK, Satishchandra P, *et al.* Characterization of human immunodeficiency virus (HIV)-infected cells in infiltrates associated with CNS opportunistic infections in patients with HIV clade C infection. *J Neuropathol Exp Neurol* 2007; **66**: 799–808.

18. Khanna N, Chandramukhi A, Desai A, *et al.* Cryptococcosis in the immunocompromised host with special reference to AIDS. *Indian J Chest Dis Allied Sci* 2000; **42**: 311–15.

19. Shankar SK, Satishchandra P, Mahadevan A, *et al.* Low prevalence of progressive multifocal leukoencephalopathy in India and Africa: is there a biological explanation? *J Neurovirol* 2003; **9**(Suppl): 59–67.

20. Holtom PD, Larsen RA, Leal ME, Leedom JM. Prevalence of neurosyphilis in human immunodeficiency virus-infected patients with latent syphilis. *Am J Med* 1992; **93**: 9–12.

21. Knopman DS, Petersen RC, Cha RH, Edland SD, Rocca WA. Incidence and causes of nondegenerative nonvascular dementia: a population based study. *Arch Neurol* 2006; **63**: 218–21.

22. Dastur DK, Lalitha VS, Udani PM, Parekh U. The brain and meninges in tuberculous meningitis-gross pathology in 100 cases and pathogenesis. *Neurol India* 1970; **18**: 86–100.

23. Treatment of tuberculosis. *MMWR* Recomm Rep 2003; **52**(RR-11):1–77.

24. Varma A, Gaur KJ. The clinical spectrum of neurocysticercosis in Uttaranchal region. *J Assoc Physicians India* 2002; **50**: 1398–400.

25. Biswas A, Prasad A, Anand KS. Cysticercal dementia. *J Assoc Physicians India* 1998; **46**: 569.

26. Mukherjee A, Roy T, Mukherjee S, *et al.* Neurocysticercosis. *J Assoc Physicians India* 1994; **42**: 87–8.

27. Ramirez-Bermudez J, Higuera J, Sosa AL, *et al.* Is dementia reversible in patients with neurocysticercosis? *J Neurol Neurosurg Psychiatry* 2005; **76**: 1164–6.

28. Forlenza OV, Filho AH, Nobrega JP, *et al.* Psychiatric manifestations of neurocysticercosis: a study of 38 patients from a neurology clinic in Brazil. *J Neurol Neurosurg Psychiatry* 1997; **62**: 612–16.

29. Satishchandra P, Shankar SK. Creutzfeldt-Jacob disease in India (1971–1990). *Neuroepidemiology* 1991; **10**: 27–32.

30. Mehndiratta MM, Bajaj BK, Gupta M, *et al.* Creutzfeldt–Jacob disease: report of 10 cases from North India. *Neurol India* 2001; **49**: 338–41.

31. Colchester AC, Colchester NT. The origin of bovine spongiform encephalopathy: the human prion disease hypothesis. *Lancet* 2005; **366**: 856–61.

32. Shankar SK, Satishchandra P. Did BSE in the UK originate from the Indian subcontinent? *Lancet* 2005; **366**: 790–1.

Cross-cultural issues of global significance

Nutrition and dementia: where is the nexus?

Alan D. Dangour and Ricardo Uauy

Introduction

There is considerable interest in the hypothesis that nutritional factors play a role in the maintenance of cognitive health in old age, and in the possibility that simple dietary modifications may alter the risk of developing cognitive impairment. The potential that this hypothesis be extended to include nutritional prevention of dementia is very appealing and frequently the subject of newspaper headlines. Indeed, recent data from Finland have suggested that dietary factors are crucial for the maintenance of cognitive health [1]. In a cohort study including more than 1400 individuals with an average age of 50 years at first examination, dementia was diagnosed in 4% of the sample at the 20-year follow-up appointment. It was also demonstrated that dementia was significantly predicted by greater age, lower education, hypertension, hypercholesterolemia, and obesity at baseline [1], clearly highlighting the consequences of good nutrition throughout the life-course for the maintenance of cognitive function.

However, while observational data seem to suggest a link between various dietary factors as diverse as curcumin [2] and vegetable juice [3], controlled clinical trials have reported mixed results when testing the efficacy of single and multinutrient dietary supplements, and other non-nutrient substances for the maintenance of cognitive function in older age [4]. In this chapter we review the strength of evidence linking micronutrients (specifically the B and antioxidant vitamins) and n-3 long-chain polyunsaturated fatty acids (n-3 LCPs) to cognitive function in older age. We also consider the implications of this evidence in the design of future studies to further elucidate the putative relationship.

Dementia: A Global Approach, ed. Ennapadam S. Krishnamoorthy, Martin J. Prince, and Jeffrey L. Cummings. Published by Cambridge University Press.

Micronutrients

A study published in 1983 which reported an association between blood levels of vitamins C and B_{12} and tests of cognitive ability among 260 free-living older people [5] was among the first to demonstrate a possible role for nutrition in cognitive health, and its findings have been confirmed on numerous occasions in the past quarter of a century. Many of these studies have focused on the potential actions of the antioxidant and B vitamins, and the accumulated evidence from cross-sectional studies is indeed quite suggestive of a link between B vitamin [6] or antioxidant vitamin status [7] and cognitive function or dementia in older people. However, establishing any measure of causality in this relationship is problematic, as clearly noted in Goodwin's original paper [5], poor diet may be both a cause and a consequence of poor cognitive function.

Furthermore, the hypothesized mechanisms by which vitamins could enhance cognitive function are complex. For example, do folate and vitamin B_{12} act directly to conserve cognitive function, or do they act by reducing the negative effects of other metabolites such as homocysteine? Folate and B_{12} status are critical modulators of plasma homocysteine concentration [8], and homocysteine is a known risk factor for the progression of atherosclerosis and altered endothelial function [9,10] which may result in brain ischemia and subsequent cognitive decline. The importance of homocysteine in this regard was demonstrated in the Rotterdam Scan study [11], which collected magnetic resonance images on 1077 individuals aged 60–90 years. This study showed that raised total homocysteine levels were significantly related to the presence of silent brain infarcts independent of other cardiovascular risk factors. Importantly, a 5-year follow-up of 1015 of these subjects demonstrated that the risk of subsequent cognitive decline was directly associated with the incidence of silent brain infarcts [12].

Given the potential importance of lowering homocysteine levels in older age, a recent trial attempted to determine whether treatment with homocysteine-lowering vitamin supplements affected cognitive performance in 276 healthy older people aged over 65 years [13]. After two years of daily supplementation with folate (1000 μg), vitamin B_{12} (500 μg) and vitamin B_6 (10 mg), or placebo, homocysteine levels were significantly reduced in the intervention arm compared to the placebo arm, but there was no effect on markers of cognitive function. The authors concluded that the trial did not support the hypothesis that lowering homocysteine results in improved cognitive performance; however, some important questions were raised in a corresponding editorial about the statistical power of the trial leaving the matter very much open for further research [14].

A recent meta-analysis, reviewing the association between plasma homocysteine levels and cardiovascular disease [15], focused on the additional risk to individuals with a mutation in a gene coding for tetrahydrofolate reductase, an enzyme involved in folate metabolism critical for its biological activity. The mutation results in a 20% elevation in plasma homocysteine levels and a concomitantly higher risk of both ischemic heart disease and deep vein thrombosis. Increasing awareness of such genetic polymorphisms commonly affecting a single nucleotide base pair of a codon, as well as the interactions between genes, known nutrients, or yet-to-be discovered food components, will likely further increase the complexity of the multiple interactions that can modulate brain function in older persons and complicate the interpretation of research in this area.

Oxidative stress has long been linked with brain aging leading many researchers to investigate a possible role for antioxidants in maintaining cognitive function. Cross-sectional surveys on this topic are common [16–19], but few studies have looked for longitudinal associations. However, a cohort study among 2889 community-dwelling adults aged 65 years and above demonstrated that individuals in the highest quintile of total vitamin E intake had a 36% lower rate of cognitive decline over 3 years of follow-up than those in the lowest vitamin E quintile [20]. While a potentially important finding, high-dose vitamin E supplementation, over 500 mg per day, has been linked to increased severity of certain morbidities [21] and increased risk of all-cause mortality [22], suggesting that dietary advice to increase vitamin E intake may be premature.

The mass of epidemiological evidence linking vitamin supplementation to cognitive function and dementia has not, however, been substantially corroborated by clinical trials in older people. Indeed a series of Cochrane reviews have concluded that there is no evidence of an effect of thiamine [23], B_6 [24], folate [25], B_{12} [24], or vitamin E [26] supplementation on cognitive health. The contradictory findings between observational and interventional studies have been discussed [27,28], and various reasons including uncontrolled confounding in observational studies, small interventions of short duration, and the unrepresentativeness of the dietary supplements used have been postulated. Numerous large trials are ongoing which will provide more information to support or refute the proposed links.

n-3 long-chain polyunsaturated fatty acids

Recent interest has focused on the possible role of n-3 LCPs, largely obtained from oily fish, in the maintenance of cognitive health. The brain is rich in the n-3 LCP docosahexaenoic acid (DHA), which, along with eicosapentaenoic acid, is known to be crucial in humans for brain development [29]. Levels of n-3 LCP in the brain fall with aging, and this has been suggested to be in part correlated with concomitant deterioration of functions of the central nervous system [30,31].

Epidemiological evidence for an association between n-3 LCP consumption and cognitive function is intriguing. One cross-sectional study reported an inverse association between fatty fish and n-3 LCP consumption and risk of cognitive impairment [32], and prospective studies have also shown inverse relationships between fish consumption and risk of dementia [32, 33] and Alzheimer's disease [34] among older people. Data from a Scottish cohort study have suggested that there may be some benefit from use of fish-oil supplements. After adjusting for childhood cognitive ability, reported daily use of fish-oil supplements was associated with improved cognitive function scores among 266 individuals aged 64 years [35]. Using a nested case-control design, this study also demonstrated that individuals reporting daily consumption of fish-oil supplements had significantly higher levels of n-3 LCPs in their erythrocyte membranes than gender-and childhood IQ-matched fish-oil supplement non-users. Furthermore, the level of total n-3 LCPs, and specifically of DHA, in erythrocyte membranes was significantly associated with cognitive ability in older age [35].

The actions of n-3 LCPs in enhancing vascular health may well provide the mechanisms for their potential role in the maintenance of cognitive health. The n-3 LCPs are known to inhibit hepatic triglyceride synthesis and, by modifying eicosanoid function, cause vascular relaxation, a diminished inflammatory process, and decreased platelet aggregation [36]. Recently, new protective actions of DHA have been discovered that may be directly related to its effects in maintaining cognitive health in older age. In a mouse model of ischemic stroke, a bioactive docosanoid derived from DHA was found to inhibit lipid peroxidation and leukocyte infiltration, which are two of the major causes of post-stroke neuronal injury [37]. This novel docosanoid, 10–17S-docosatriene, now called neuroprotectin D1 [38], potently down-regulates proinflammatory gene expression in cultured neuronal cells [37]. Docosahexaenoic acid also protects in vitro cultured hippocampal neurons from apoptosis (programmed cell death) [39], potentially via the ability of neuroprotectin D1 to counteract oxidative-stress triggered DNA damage, as well as up-regulate antiapoptotic, and down-regulate proapoptotic, protein expression [38].

Again, however, the epidemiological and mechanistic evidence is not supported by data from randomized trials, and a recent Cochrane review was unable to locate a single published trial on which to base recommendations for the use of dietary or supplemental n-3 LCPs for the prevention of cognitive impairment or dementia [28]. The recently published OPAL study, which aimed to determine the effect of daily n-3 LCP supplementation on cognitive function in healthy older people, was unable to detect an effect of supplementation over 2 years [40].

Conclusions

Despite considerable research effort over the past 25 years, there is still a lack of good quality evidence to identify which dietary factors are able to help maintain cognitive health in older age. It is likely that sufficiency in B and antioxidant vitamins is important, and there is equally some evidence to support the hypothesized role for n-3 LCPs, but randomized trial evidence is lacking. A recent call for meta-analysis of large trials of the actions of B vitamins on cardiovascular health may also provide information on the relevance of B vitamins for the maintenance of cognitive function [41], but better designed and larger sample size trials are also needed.

Perhaps the last word should go to Murray Raskind who wrote an editorial on Goodwin's original paper. When referring to the lack of success of trials Raskind stated "Although this should not discourage further research on the relationship between nutrition and cognitive function, it does underscore the critical importance of rigorous experimental design if such studies are to be meaningfully interpreted, and it suggests that nutritional supplementation cannot yet be viewed as a demonstrably effective therapy for cognitive problems in the elderly" [42].

References

1. Kivipelto M, Ngandu T, Laatikainen T, *et al.* Risk score for the prediction of dementia risk in 20 years among middle aged people: a longitudinal, population-based study. *Lancet Neurol* 2006; **5**(9): 735–41.
2. Ng TP, Chiam PC, Lee T, *et al.* Curry consumption and cognitive function in the elderly. *Am J Epidemiol* 2006; **164**(9): 898–906.
3. Dai Q, Borenstein AR, Wu Y, Jackson JC, Larson EB. Fruit and vegetable juices and Alzheimer's disease: the Kame Project. *Am J Med* 2006; **119**(9): 751–9.
4. Manders M, de Groot LC, Van Staveren WA, *et al.* Effectiveness of nutritional supplements on cognitive functioning in elderly persons: a systematic review. *J Gerontol A Biol Sci Med Sci* 2004; **59**(10): 1041–9.
5. Goodwin JS, Goodwin JM, Garry PJ. Association between nutritional status and cognitive functioning in a healthy elderly population. *JAMA* 1983; **249**(21): 2917–21.
6. Selhub J, Bagley LC, Miller J, Rosenberg IH. B vitamins, homocysteine, and neurocognitive function in the elderly. *Am J Clin Nutr* 2000; **71**(2): 614S-20S.
7. Frank B, Gupta S. A review of antioxidants and Alzheimer's disease. *Ann Clin Psychiatry* 2005; **17**(4): 269–86.
8. Selhub J, Miller JW The pathogenesis of homocysteinemia: interruption of the coordinate regulation by S-adenosylmethionine of the remethylation and transsulfuration of homocysteine. *Am J Clin Nutr* 1992; **55**(1): 131–8.
9. Boushey CJ, Beresford SA, Omenn GS, Motulsky AG. A quantitative assessment of plasma homocysteine as a risk factor for vascular disease. Probable benefits of increasing folic acid intakes. *JAMA* 1995; **274**(13): 1049–57.
10. Hankey GJ, Eikelboom JW. Homocysteine and vascular disease. *Lancet* 1999; **354**(9176): 407–13.
11. Vermeer SE, van Dijk EJ, Koudstaal PJ, *et al.* Homocysteine, silent brain infarcts, and white matter lesions: The Rotterdam Scan Study. *Ann Neurol* 2002; **51**(3): 285–9.
12. Vermeer SE, Prins ND, den Heijer T, *et al.* Silent brain infarcts and the risk of dementia and cognitive decline. *N Engl J Med* 2003; **348**(13): 1215–22.
13. McMahon JA, Green TJ, Skeaff CM *et al.* A controlled trial of homocysteine lowering and cognitive performance. *N Engl J Med* 2006; **354**(26): 2764–72.
14. Clarke, R. Vitamin B12, folic acid, and the prevention of dementia. *N Engl J Med* 2006; **354**(26): 2817–19.
15. Wald DS, Law M, Morris JK. Homocysteine and cardiovascular disease: evidence on causality from a meta-analysis. *BMJ* 2002; **325**(7374): 1202.
16. Haller J, Weggemans RM, Ferry M, Guigoz Y. Mental health: minimental state examination and geriatric depression score of elderly Europeans in the SENECA study of 1993. *Eur J Clin Nutr* 1996; **50** (Suppl 2): S112–16.
17. Jama JW, Launer LJ, Witteman JC, *et al.* Dietary antioxidants and cognitive function in a population-based sample of older persons. The Rotterdam Study. *Am J Epidemiol* 1996 **144**(3): 275–80.
18. Perrig WJ, Perrig P, Stähelin HB. The relation between antioxidants and memory performance in the old and very old. *J Am Geriatr Soc* 1997; **45**(6): 718–24.
19. Perkins AJ, Hendrie HC, Callahan CM, *et al.* Association of antioxidants with memory in

a multiethnic elderly sample using the Third National Health and Nutrition Examination Survey. *Am J Epidemiol* 1999; **150**(1): 37–44.

20. Morris MC, Evans DA, Bienias JL, Tangney CC, Wilson RS. Vitamin E and cognitive decline in older persons. *Arch Neurol* 2002; **59**(7): 1125–32.
21. Graat JM, Schouten EG, Kok FJ. Effect of daily vitamin E and multivitamin-mineral supplementation on acute respiratory tract infections in elderly persons: a randomized controlled trial. *JAMA* 2002; **288**(6): 715–21.
22. Miller ER 3rd, Pastor-Barriuso R, Dalal D, *et al.* Meta-analysis: high-dosage vitamin E supplementation may increase all-cause mortality. *Ann Intern Med* 2005; **142**(1): 37–46.
23. Rodriguez-Martin JL, Qizilbash N, López-Arrieta JM. Thiamine for Alzheimer's disease. *Cochrane Database Syst Rev* 2001; (2): CD001498.
24. Malouf R, Grimley EJ. The effect of vitamin B6 on cognition. *Cochrane Database Syst Rev* 2003; (4): CD004393.
25. Malouf M, Grimley EJ, Areosa SA. Folic acid with or without vitamin B12 for cognition and dementia. *Cochrane Database Syst Rev* 2003; (4): CD004514.
26. Tabet N, Birks J, Grimley Evans J. Vitamin E for Alzheimer's disease *(Cochrane Review) Issue 1.* Oxford, Update Software, 2003.
27. Lawlor DA, Davey Smith G, Kundu D, Bruckdorfer KR, Ebrahim S. Those confounded vitamins: what can we learn from the differences between observational versus randomized trial evidence? *Lancet* 2004; **363**(9422): 1724–7.
28. Lim WS, Gammack JK, Van Nieker KJ, Dangour AD. Omega 3 fatty acid for the prevention of dementia. *Cochrane Database Syst Rev* 2006; (1): CD005379.
29. Uauy R, Hoffman DR, Peirano P, Birch DG, Birch EE. Essential fatty acids in visual and brain development. *Lipids* 2001; **36**(9): 885–95.
30. Söderberg M, Edlund C, Kristensson K, Dallner G. Lipid compositions of different regions of the human brain during aging. *J Neurochem* 1990; **54**(2): 415–23.
31. Soderberg M, Edlund C, Kristersson K, Dallner G. Fatty acid composition of brain phospholipids in aging and in Alzheimer's disease. *Lipids* 1991; **26**(6): 421–5.
32. Kalmijn S, Feskens EJ, Launer LJ, Kromhout D. Polyunsaturated fatty acids, antioxidants, and cognitive function in very old men. *Am J Epidemiol* 1997; **145**(1): 33–41.
33. Barberger-Gateau P, Letenneur L, Deschamps v, *et al.* Fish, meat, and risk of dementia: cohort study. *BMJ* 2002; **325**(7370): 932–3.
34. Morris MC, Evans DA, Bienias JL, *et al.* Consumption of fish and n-3 fatty acids and risk of incident Alzheimer disease. *Arch Neurol* 2003; **60**(7): 940–6.
35. Duthie SJ, Whalley LJ, Collins AR, *et al.* Homocysteine, B vitamin status, and cognitive function in the elderly. *Am J Clin Nutr* 2002; **75**(5): 908–13.
36. Uauy R, Valenzuela A. Marine oils: the health benefits of n-3 fatty acids. *Nutrition* 2000; **16**(7–8): 680–4.
37. Marcheselli VL, Hong S, Lukiw WJ, *et al.* Novel docosanoids inhibit brain ischemia-reperfusion-mediated leukocyte infiltration and pro-inflammatory gene expression. *J Biol Chem* 2003; **278**(44): 43807–17.
38. Mukherjee PK, Marcheselli VL, Serhan CN, Bazan NG. Neuroprotectin D1: a docosahexaenoic acid-derived docosatriene protects human retinal pigment epithelial cells

from oxidative stress. *Proc Natl Acad Sci U S A* 2004; **101**(22): 8491–6.

39. Kim HY, Akbar M, Lau A, Edsall L. Inhibition of neuronal apoptosis by docosahexaenoic acid (22:6n-3). Role of phosphatidylserine in antiapoptotic effect. *J Biol Chem* 2000; **275**(45): 35215–23.

40. Dangour AD, Allen LH, Elbourne D, *et al.* Effect of 2-y n-3 long-chain polyunsaturated fatty acid supplementation on cognitive function in older people: a randomized, double-blind, controlled trial. *Am J Clin Nutr* 2010; **91**(6): 1725–32.

41. B-vitamin Treatment Trialists Collaboration. Homocysteine-lowering trials for prevention of cardiovascular events: a review of the design and power of the large randomized trials. *Am Heart J* 2006; **151**(2): 282–7.

42. Raskind M. Nutrition and cognitive function in the elderly. *JAMA* 1983; **249**(21): 2939–40.

Assessment

The experience of assessing cognition across cultures

Kathleen S. Hall

A consensus of thought about the possible causes of Alzheimer's disease and mild cognitive impairment is mushrooming among scientists throughout the world. There is agreement in various degrees that the development of disease probably involves a complex interaction of genetic and environmentally influenced factors [1,2]. The puzzle of unraveling these factors and their possible mechanisms can be significantly enhanced if we can compare the patterns of distribution of disease and the presence or absence of putative risk factors in populations living in quite different environments [3,4]. Comparative studies offer enormous challenges to investigators. Such studies require rigorous adherence to methods which will ensure that the data produced in diverse settings will indeed be scientifically comparable. If comparative studies are to live up to the promise they hold for science, they must unequivocally yield data that will allow comparisons of "apples to apples." The focus of this chapter is the assessment of cognition at the community screening level rather than in a clinical diagnostic level. This means that the cognitive assessment is given to individuals living in the community whom we invite to participate in a study, as opposed to motivated individuals bringing a complaint to a clinic for diagnosis and treatment.

The assessment of cognition of interest for this chapter is determined by the criteria we use to diagnose dementia and Alzheimer's disease. The most generally used criteria for the diagnosis of dementia are those of the Diagnostic and Statistical Manual of Mental Disorders published by the American Psychiatric Association, DSM III-R [5], and DSM IV-TR [6]. For diagnosing Alzheimer's disease the criteria proposed by the National Institute of Neurological and Communicative Diseases and Stroke/Alzheimer's Disease and Related Disorders Association (NINCDS/ADRDA) [7] are the standard. A milder form of cognitive

Dementia: A Global Approach, ed. Ennapadam S. Krishnamoorthy, Martin J. Prince, and Jeffrey L. Cummings. Published by Cambridge University Press.

impairment is of interest to researchers because some such cases may be preclinical Alzheimer's disease that do go on to fully develop dementia, while others either get better or remain mildly impaired for years. Criteria for this milder form of impairment are currently hotly debated in the literature as evidence accrues [8–14]. Due to the current lack of consensus on the diagnostic criteria and difficulties inherent in assessment of subtleties of minor cognitive decline, assessment of mild cognitive impairment will not be addressed in this chapter.

In our quest to determine rates and risk factors for age-associated dementias throughout the globe, we must give careful consideration to our methods of case ascertainment. Cognitive tests are notoriously influenced by level of education, while other cultural and environmental factors may also influence test performance. International comparative studies of rates and risk factors hold promise for testing hypotheses regarding the etiology of disease; however, great care must be taken in order to construct studies that are truly comparable. While the research designs for epidemiological studies may be fairly adaptable for application among various countries and cultures, the diagnostic assessments must be carefully crafted to accommodate the prevailing conditions of each language and culture. Evaluation of cognitive function is a delicate task regardless of objective, and the evaluation of decline in the elderly can be even more of a challenge except in the case of longitudinal studies in which decline can actually be measured. Such longitudinal studies are expensive and carry their own unique methodological problems but remain the ideal design for epidemiological studies.

Our research group at Indiana University has collaborated with researchers at the University of Ibadan, Nigeria on a comparative epidemiological study of rates and risk factors for Alzheimer's disease since 1992. This community-based longitudinal study reported significantly lower incidence rates for the Yoruba compared to African Americans [15]. We are conducting studies of putative risk factors, both environmental and genetic, that may explain these differences in rates. One important finding has been that apolipoprotein E e4 (*APOE4*) is a risk factor in the African Americans [16] but is not associated with the disease in the Yoruba [17]. The African Americans have higher rates of cholesterolemia than the Yoruba, and there is an interaction between *APOE4*, cholesterol level, and risk for Alzheimer's disease in both populations [2] (see Chapter 3 for other comparative perspectives). Our groups continue to follow these two well-characterized cohorts to test emerging hypotheses of etiology of disease.

In order to select the most appropriate method of assessment one must be quite clear about the purpose of the test. The studies conducted by our research group in sites in various countries have followed a two-stage design. In the first screening stage, we administer the Community Screening Interview for Dementia (CSI-D) to all subjects in the representative community-based sample. This also includes an interview with a close relative regarding the primary subject's activities of daily living, comparing current functioning to past level of functioning. On the basis of performance on the CSI-D individuals are selected for a second stage in which a full standardized clinical assessment is carried out including the following: (1) neuropsychological tests (following the Consortium to Establish a Registry for Alzheimer's Disease; CERAD) [18,19]; (2) standardized physical and neurological examination and functional status review [20]; (3) semi-structured interview with a relative; and (4) request for medical records. We will focus here upon the screening interview.

The purpose of the screening interview is to identify individuals who have the greatest probability of being demented although, in our studies, we also carry out the full clinical assessment on a sample of individuals who do well on the CSI-D to test for false negatives. The CSI-D is an interview administered at a single point in time and therefore only represents the subject's current cognitive status. The hallmark symptom of dementia is decline in cognitive function and to assess possibility of such change the CSI-D includes an interview with a close relative. The CSI-D includes items to test domains of cognition comprising the criteria for diagnosis of the DSM-III-R as well as DSM-IV-TR. The CSI-D takes about 30 minutes and includes items to test the following domains of cognitive function: short- and long-term memory, abstract thinking, judgment, higher cortical function – aphasia, agnosia, apraxia, and constructional ability. The interview with the relative provides data on whether cognitive deficits are severe enough to cause impairment in social or occupational functioning.

The CSI-D was first developed by our group for a study of Cree Indians in Manitoba, Canada, for comparison to non-Indian Canadians living in Winnipeg [21]. In subsequent studies we worked with local colleagues to adapt it for use in African Americans, Yoruba of Nigeria [22], Jamaicans, Kenyans, and Chinese. In each of the studies described here for which the CSI-D was translated, analyses of sensitivity, specificity, and area under the receiver operating characteristic (ROC) curve were conducted to examine the effectiveness of the instrument to discriminate demented from not demented study participants. Comparisons of data from the various sites were previously published, and demonstrated the effectiveness to identify dementia and the adaptability of the instrument for diverse languages and cultures [23].

The 10/66 Dementia Research Group, a consortium of researchers from various parts of the world, has used a one-stage design for epidemiological studies in developing countries. The Group conducted pilot studies in 25 centers in India, China, Southeast Asia, Latin America, the Caribbean, and Africa using translated and harmonized versions of well-established instruments. The CSI-D was used, with the animal fluency item scored separately, in combination with the CERAD ten-word list learning task [24] and the Geriatric Mental State/Automated Geriatric Examination for Computer Assisted Taxonomy (GMS/AGECAT) [25]. The 10/66 studies developed an algorithm combining data from each of the instruments for diagnosis of dementia that proved to work better than any of the instruments alone [26].

In each site in which the CSI-D has been used by our group, the individual items are first evaluated and translated to adapt to the language and culture in which it will be used. This process is carried out by members of our interdisciplinary research team in collaboration with researchers who are also native speakers. Items are also "harmonized," a process that insures the question will be harmonious with the language and culture as well as the age cohort to be tested. The objective of the harmonization process is to avoid wording of questions that might offend, mislead, insult, or otherwise detract from the test. The experience of our research group has revealed nuances of grammar that may be acceptable in younger people but considered disrespectful by elderly in the same population. One glaring example of this would be rap-type slang used by young American Blacks, but considered vulgar by the elderly. Our group found such age cohort effects in each of the cultures we studied.

The translation process takes time and patience as well as several iterations before a pilot test can be conducted for a new target population. Figure 6A.1 shows the recommended steps in the adaptation of the CSI-D for a new language or culture. Items are independently translated, and back translated and tested with small samples of elderly for acceptability, followed by a formal pilot study to establish normative values and cutoff scores.

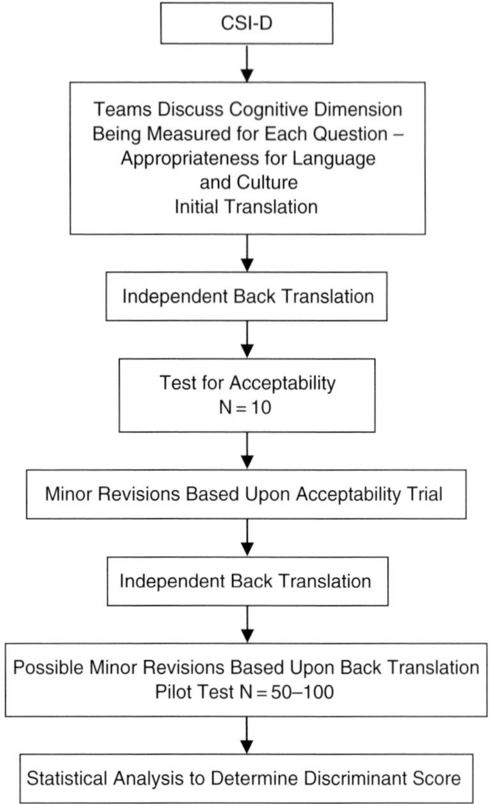

Figure 6A.1 The recommended steps in the adaptation of CSI-D for a new language or culture.

During the course of initially constructing the CSI-D and subsequently adapting it for additional languages, our group made a few significant changes to traditional psychometric methods. One notable example is the testing of the ability to name objects. Traditional tests show the subject either a drawing or photograph of the target object. For the CSI-D we point to actual objects. The objects to be named are with the interviewer: pencil, shoes, watch, chair, elbow, knuckles, and shoulder. This technique may be especially adaptable when the subject has sensory deficits such as hearing or visual impairment, in which case the interviewer can have the subject touch the object, and the interviewer can indicate the body part on the subject.

Some of the CSI-D items have proven to be usable with fairly straightforward translation; these are presented in Table 6A.1. One of the memory tests of the CSI-D asks the subject to remember the interviewer's name. Since the interviewers are local residents, this item easily adapts to the local conditions. The memory item using three words – boat, house, fish – has worked well in each translation. The language comprehension – motor response items – have also been translated with very little change in various languages: 1. Please nod your

Table 6A.1 Questions that are the same in the different languages

Cognitive items Memory:	Remember my name: ("I'd like you to remember my name. My last name is _____. Can you repeat that, please? I want you to remember it because I will ask you my name a little later.") Remember 3 words: boat, house, fish Repeat story: Three children were alone at home and the house caught on fire. A brave man managed to climb in a back window and carry them to safety. Aside from minor cuts and bruises, all were well. Repeat story again after constructional items	
Abstract thinking	What is a bridge?	What do people do in church/ mosque?
	What do you do with a hammer?	Where do we go to buy medicine?
Higher cortical function	Name these items as I point to them: pencil, watch, chair, shoes, knuckles, elbow, + shoulder	
	Name as many animals as possible in one minute.	
Language comprehension	Please nod your head. Point first to the window, then to the door.	Take paper in right hand, fold in half, put in lap
Construction ability		
Orientation/Time	Month, Day, Year, Season	

head. 2. Please point first to the window then to the door (applicable whether the interview is conducted inside or outside of the home). 3. I am going to give you a piece of paper. When I do, take the paper in your right hand, fold the paper in half with both hands, and put the paper down on your lap.

Assessment of orientation to place employs items that must be very specific for each study site; examples are given in Table 6A.2. In areas where formal addresses are not used, we have adapted the local systems for geographic orientation such as proximity to well-known landmarks: a body of water, main road, or gathering place. The long-term memory items also are site specific, and ask about commonly recognized historical figures or events. There is also a language item that asks the study participant to repeat a well-known idiomatic phrase. By this, we mean a commonly used phrase that means something beyond a literal translation. The English phrase "no ifs, ands, or buts" is commonly used by parents to emphasize a "no" response to their children, stressing there is no ambiguity about the topic in question. The Yoruba phrase "Oke gb'oke g'ope" translates

Table 6A.2 Questions that differ among languages

Orientation/ place	What is the name of this city/village/town/ reserve? What is the name of the mayor/chief?	Where is the local market/bay store? What is your address/who lives next door?
	What are the names of two major streets near here/is the part of the reserve we are in/is the name of a river near here?	
Language	"Now I would like for you to repeat what I say: 'No ifs, ands, or buts.'" 'Kit tit taw na mana.' 'Oke gb'oke g'ope.' (Phrases are idiomatic in each language.)	
Long-term memory	USA: What is the name of the civil rights leader who was assassinated in Memphis in 1968? Nigeria: Who was the military leader of the Ibos during the Nigerian civil war fought from 1967 to 1970? China: Who established the New China? Jamaica: Who was Nanny?	

to "Oke carried a sack up a palm tree"; however, beyond this literal meaning it is a well-known tongue twister, with the side benefit of often evoking a smile from the study participant.

The CSI-D includes an interview with a close relative about the daily functioning of the primary study participant. Table 6A.3 lists the items of the relative interview that have proven to require very little adaptation for various languages in spite of wide variation in living conditions. There are two important reasons to interview a relative. First, the relative is able to provide information on the subject's current functioning compared to earlier functioning for evidence of cognitive decline. This evidence also addresses one of the criteria for dementia having to do with whether the severity of cognitive deficits is sufficient to cause impairment in social or occupational functioning. Second, there is a very low correlation between education level and scores on the interview with the relative, which helps to attenuate possible confounding of dementia with effects of low education for the cognitive score. Although the CSI-D was designed for use in illiterate as well as literate populations, the effects of education have not been entirely overcome. Our group recently examined the assessment of cognitive function by the relative by comparing it to actual cognitive scores for a test of validity, and found significant correlations cross-sectionally as well as in a five-year follow-up [27]. The score from the interview with the relative is combined with the cognitive score of the CSI-D to yield a discriminant score, which separates the demented and the not demented subjects better than the cognitive score alone [22].

Table 6A.3 Interview with close relative: items the same in different languages

Memory and cognition	Remembering is a problem Forgets where he/she puts things Forgets where things are usually kept Forgets names of friends Forgets names of members of the family Forgets what wanted to say in mid-conversation	Forgets when last saw you Forgets what happened the day before Forgets where he/she is Gets lost in the community Gets lost in own home
Activities of daily living (ADL)	Difficulty with: household tasks, adjusting to change, feeding self, dressing, using toilet Change in ability to handle money	Loss of skill or hobby Change in ability to think and reason
Miscellaneous problems	Change in activities Decline in mental functioning	Difficulty finding right word

This chapter presented the rationale and the process for adapting the CSI-D for use in a different language and culture. It has been shown to reliably and validly discriminate between demented and not demented community-dwelling samples in different languages and cultures. It should be noted that it was developed and has been used by our research groups as a screening instrument for studies employing a two-stage study design. It can also be effectively used for one-stage studies when combined with other instruments, as demonstrated by the work of the 10/66 Dementia Research Group. Although efforts were made to reduce the effect of education on the cognitive score, a small significant correlation must be recognized and taken into consideration if the CSI-D is employed. This screening interview has proven to be adaptable but must be carefully harmonized and translated as well as pilot tested before using it in a new target population in order to establish appropriate normative values and cut off scores.

Acknowledgments

NIH/NIA Grant #RO1-AG09956–15

Francine L. Bray and Jenna L. York for technical support.

References

1. Lahiri DK, Sambamurti K, Bennett DA. Apolipoprotein gene and its interaction with the environmentally driven risk factors: molecular, genetic and epidemiological studies of Alzheimer's disease. *Neurobiol Aging* 2004; **25**(5): 651–60.
2. Hall KS, Murrell J, Ogunniyi A, *et al.* Cholesterol, APOE genotype and Alzheimer's disease: an epidemiological study of Nigerian Yoruba. *Neurology* 2006; **66**: 223–7.

3. Hendrie HC, Murrell J, Gao S, *et al.* International studies in dementia with particular emphasis on populations of African origin. *Alzheimer Dis Assoc Disord* 2006; **20**(3 Suppl 2): S42–6.
4. Prince M, Graham N, Brodaty H, *et al.* Alzheimer Disease International's 10/66 Dementia Research Group-One model for action research in developing countries. *Int J Geriatr Psychiatry* 2004; **19**: 178–81.
5. American Psychiatric Association. *Diagnostic and Statistical Manual of Mental Disorders*, 3rd edn., Revised. Washington, DC, American Psychiatric Association, 1987.
6. American Psychiatric Association. *Diagnostic and Statistical Manual of Mental Disorders, Fourth Edition, Text Revision (DSM-IV-TR).* Washington, DC, American Psychiatric Association Press, 2000.
7. McKhann G, Drachman D, Folstein M, *et al.* Clinical diagnosis of Alzheimer's disease: Report of the NINCDS-ADRDA Work Group under the auspices of the Department of Health and Human Services Task Force on Alzheimer's Disease. *Neurology* 1984; **34**(7): 939–44.
8. Petersen RC, Doody R, Kurz A, *et al.* Current concepts in mild cognitive impairment. *Arch Neurol* 2001; **58**(12): 1985–1992.
9. Petersen R. Mild cognitive impairment as a diagnostic entity. *J Intern Med* 2004; **156**: 183–94.
10. Smith GE, Petersen RC, Parisi JE, *et al.* Definition, course, and outcome of mild cognitive impairment. *Aging Neuropsychol Cogn* 1996; **3**: 131–47.
11. Morris JC, Storandt M, Miller JP, *et al.* Mild cognitive impairment represents early-stage Alzheimer disease. *Arch Neurol* 2001; **58**(3): 397–405.
12. Morris JC, McKeel DW Jr, *et al.* Very mild Alzheimer's disease: informant-based clinical, psychometric, and pathologic distinction from normal aging. *Neurology* 1991; **41**(4): 469–78.
13. Ritchie K, Artero S, Touchon J. Classification criteria for mild cognitive impairment: a population-based validation study. *Neurology* 2001; **56**(1): 37–42.
14. Ritchie K, Touchon J. Mild cognitive impairment: conceptual basis and current nosological status. *Lancet* 2000; **355**(9199): 225–8.
15. Hendrie HC, Gao S, Murray MD, Hall KS, Richards SS. In Reply to: Gambassi G, Onder G and Bernabei R. In re hypertension and cognition: enough to be confused. *J Am Geriatr Soc* 2001; **49**(6): 840–1.
16. Murrell JR, Price B, Lane KA, *et al.* Association of apolipoprotein E genotype and Alzheimer disease in African Americans. *Arch Neurol* 2006; **63**: 431–4.
17. Gureje O, Ogunniyi A, Baiyewu O, *et al. APOE* 4 is not associated with Alzheimer's disease in elderly Nigerians. *Ann Neurol* 2006; **59**(1): 182–5.
18. Unverzagt FW, Hall KS, Torke AM, *et al.* Effects of age, education, and gender on CERAD neuropsychological test performance in an African American sample. *Clin Neuropsychol* 1996; **10**(2): 180–90.
19. Gureje O, Unverzagt FW, Osuntokun BO, *et al.* The CERAD neuropsychological test battery: norms from a Yoruba-speaking Nigerian sample. *West Afr J Med* 1995; **14**(1): 29–33.
20. Hendrie HC, Lane KA, Ogunniyi A, *et al.* The development of a semi-structured home interview (CHIF) to directly assess function in cognitively impaired elderly people in two cultures. *Int Psychogeriatr* 2006; **18**(4): 653–66.

21. Hall KS, Hendrie HC, Brittain HM, Prince CS, Rodgers DD. Community Screening Interview for Dementia (CSI"D"). Nelson House Cree Version Collaborative Epidemiology Study. *Int J Methods Psychiatr Res* 1993; **3**: 15–28.

22. Hall KS, Ogunniyi AO, Hendrie HC, *et al.* A cross-cultural community based study of dementias: methods and performance of the survey instrument, Indianapolis, U.S.A., and Ibadan, Nigeria. *Int J Methods Psychiatr Res* 1996; **6**: 129–42.

23. Hall KS, Gao S, Emsley CL, *et al.* Community Screening Interview for Dementia (CSI"D"): performance in five disparate study sites. *Int J Geriatr Psychiatry* 2000; **15**(6): 521–31.

24. Morris JC, Mohs RC, Rogers H, Fillenbaum G, Heyman A. Consortium to establish a registry for Alzheimer's disease (CERAD) clinical and neuropsychological assessment of Alzheimer's disease. *Psychopharmacol Bull* 1988; **24**: 641–52.

25. Copeland JRM, Dewey ME, Griffith-Jones HM. A computerised psychiatric diagnostic system and case nomenclature for elderly subjects: GMS and AGECAT. *Psychol Med* 1986; **16**: 89–99.

26. Prince M, Acosta D, Chiu H, Scazufca M, Varghese M. 10/66 Dementia Research Group. Dementia diagnosis in developing countries: a cross-cultural validation study. *Lancet* 2003; **361**(9361): 909–17.

27. Shen J, Gao S, Unverzagt FW, *et al.* Validation analysis of informant's ratings of cognitive function in African Americans and Nigerians. *Int J Geriatr Psychiatry* 2006; **21**: 1–8.

Assessment

Assessing behavior in dementia across cultures

Vorapun Senanarong and Jeffrey L. Cummings

Introduction

Dementia is characterized by cognitive impairment, functional decline, and presence of behavioral and neuropsychiatric symptoms. However, the presence of neuropsychiatric symptoms is not required for a diagnosis of dementia. Only dementia with Lewy bodies and frontotemporal lobar dementia include behavioral and neuropsychiatric symptoms in their definition of diseases. Behavioral and neuropsychiatric symptoms in patients of dementia are increasingly recognized as being important as determinants of patient distress, caregiver burden, quality of life of both patients and caregivers, and outcome of dementia. The frequency and severity of neuropsychiatric disturbances increase in late stage of dementia [1].

It is noteworthy that the prevalence and tolerability of some behavioral and psychological symptoms of dementia (BPSD) depend on environmental, educational, and cultural backgrounds. Apathy is more commonly reported in American than in Chinese patients [2] while wandering and shouting are more tolerated in Australian than in Chinese nursing homes [3].

Terminology and definition

Various terminologies have been used to describe and encapsulate behavioral and neuropsychiatric features in dementia. The term BPSD is commonly used to refer to a heterogeneous collection of psychological problems, psychiatric symptoms, and behavioral alterations in patients with dementia of any cause [4]. The psychological symptoms in BPSD include delusions, hallucinations, misidentification, depression, sleeplessness, and anxiety. Behavioral symptoms in BPSD include physical aggression, wandering, and restlessness. Behavioral and psychological symptoms of dementia include common symptoms that cause distress, and symptoms that are likely manageable (Table 6B.1). The Behavioral

Dementia: A Global Approach, ed. Ennapadam S. Krishnamoorthy, Martin J. Prince, and Jeffrey L. Cummings. Published by Cambridge University Press.

Table 6B.1 Comparison of behavioral symptoms included in the Behavioral Pathology in Alzheimer's Disease Rating Scale (BEHAVE-AD), Behavioral and Psychological Symptoms of Dementia (BPSD), Behavioral Rating Scale for Dementia (BRSD), and Neuropsychiatric Inventory (NPI)

BEHAVE-AD	*BPSD*	*BRSD*	*NPI*
Paranoid/delusional ideation; hallucinations	Psychological symptoms of :	Psychotic symptoms	Delusions
	Delusions		Hallucinations
	Hallucinations		
	Misidentifications		
Affective disturbances	Depression	Depressive symptoms	Depression, dysphoria
Diurnal rhythm disturbances	Sleeplessness	Inertia	Night-time behaviors
Anxieties and phobias	Anxiety		Anxiety
	Behavioral symptoms of:		
Aggressiveness	Physical aggression	Aggression	Agitation/ aggression
Activity disturbances	Wandering		Aberrant motor behavior
	Restlessness	Irritability	Irritability
	Other common BPSD include agitation, culturally inappropriate behavior, pacing, screaming		Disinhibition
	Manageable BPSD that are less likely to lead to institutionalization: crying, cursing, apathy, repetitive questioning, shadowing		Apathy, indifference
		Vegetative symptoms	Appetite/eating behaviors
			Elation/euphoria

Rating Scale for Dementia (BRSD) [5] is based on the caregiver's report on the presence or frequency of 46 behaviors that can be grouped into 6 subscales: depression, inertia, vegetative symptoms, irritability and aggression, behavioral dysregulation, and psychotic symptoms. The Behavioral Pathology in Alzheimer Disease Rating Scale (BEHAVE-AD) [6] is the assessment that obtains information from caregivers to rate 25 behavioral symptoms. Symptoms in BEHAVE-AD can be clustered into seven groups: paranoid and delusional ideation, hallucinations, aggressiveness, activity disturbances, diurnal rhythm disturbances, affective disturbances, and anxieties and phobias. The Neuropsychiatric Inventory (NPI) [7] looks at caregiver rating on frequency and severity of 12 specific behaviors. Comparison of these scales is shown in Table 6B.1. Each of these measures has proven to be validated for dementia and reliable to use. It is worth noticing that BEHAVE-AD has a global rating, NPI has a summary score, and BRSD has factors scores. They are multiple-domain-specific tools to assess behavioral and neuropsychiatric problems in patients with dementia. The BEHAVE-AD and NPI are among the most commonly used multi-domain behavioral assessment tools in many countries both in Asia and in the West, in the clinic setting and in clinical trials. Suh and Kim [8] reported that 92% of 562 antipsychotic naïve Alzheimer's disease (AD) patients from four different groups in Korea (a geriatric mental hospital, a semi-hospitalized dementia institute, a dementia clinic, and community-dwelling dementia patients) had at least one BPSD assessed by the BEHAVE-AD. Fifty-six percent had four or more BPSD. Behavioral disturbances peak at the stages of moderate or moderate-severe AD. Alzheimer's disease patients left at home without treatment had higher frequency of BPSD than those seeking active treatment, although all of them were antipsychotic-naïve. Fuh *et al.* [9] described neuropsychiatric manifestations in patients with AD, and cortical and subcortical vascular dementia (VaD) in Taiwan using the NPI. Of the 536 patients with dementia, cortical VaD patients had the highest mean composite NPI scores in all domains and AD patients had the lowest mean composite scores in most domains.

There are a number of single-domain assessments focused on specific behavioral dysfunction. Commonly known measures are Agitated Behavior Inventory for Dementia, Cohen-Mansfield Agitation Inventory, Overt Aggression Scale, Apathy Scale, Cornell Scale for Depression in Dementia, Geriatric Depression Scale, Hamilton Rating Scale for Depression, Hamilton Rating Scale for Anxiety, Irritability Scale, or Positive and Negative Syndrome Scale [10].

Apart from the aforementioned transcultural and disease-type differences, it is interesting to note that studies from community-based populations have revealed in general a lower frequency of BPSD when compared with clinic-based reports.

Descriptions of specific behavioral symptoms and their cross-cultural implications

Depression

Depression in AD defined by the National Institute of Mental Health (NIMH-dAD) [11] requires only three depressive symptoms out of nine symptoms from Diagnostic and Statistical Manual of Mental Disorders, fourth edition (DSM-IV) criteria [12] for major depression. Duration and frequency of depressive symptoms in AD need be present together within the same 2-week period, as compared with DSM-IV prerequisite that symptoms occur most of the day, nearly every day, for at least 2 weeks. The decreased ability to think and concentrate previously included here, was removed, due to poor specificity in AD. The criteria for anhedonia in AD focus on decreased affect and pleasure associated with social and other activities. Social withdrawal and irritability were added in this population. The NIMH-dAD criteria exhibited 94% sensitivity and 85% specificity [13]. However, in Starkstein and coworkers' report [14], it was found that when patients were diagnosed with the NIMH criteria (i.e., depressed mood or loss of positive affect and at least three additional symptoms of depression), 41% of depressed patients in the stage of severe AD had no sad mood, suggesting that the NIMH criteria may have low specificity for depression in the late stages of dementia.

The relationship between AD and late-onset depression is complex. Major depression, which affects about 25% of patients with AD, has major consequences both for the patients themselves and for caregivers [15]. The relationship between AD and depression burden or distress in the caregiver may depend on the cultural background. Pang *et al.* [16] looked at the effect of depression and apathy on caregiver distress in American Chinese caregivers and Caucasian American caregivers. They reported that Chinese caregivers were less affected by depression and apathy in patients with AD than Caucasian caregivers.

Apathy and other motivational syndromes

Apathy is reported in high frequency in patients with stroke, Parkinson's disease, AD, and traumatic brain injury [17]. Disorders of diminished motivation include apathy, abulia, akinetic mutism, Kluver–Bucy syndrome, emotional indifference, negative symptoms schizophrenia, and anergia. Apathy is defined as the absence or lack of feeling, emotion, interest, concern, or motivation not attributable to decreased level of consciousness, cognitive impairment, or emotional disturbance [18] (Table 6B.2). Levy and Dubois [19] recently suggested that apathy is an observable behavioral syndrome consisting of a quantitative reduction of self-generated voluntary and purposeful behavioral change relative to the previous behavioral pattern of the individual and absence of contextual or physical changes. A recent report from an international workshop on neuropsychiatric manifestation in Asia stated that apathy is more difficult to detect and characterize in Asian populations [20]. Apathy is not depression. Some reports found prevalence of apathy of 37% in AD [17], compared to none in healthy subjects. In 24% of the AD sample, apathy coexisted with dysthymic disorder or major depression, but 13% had apathy without depression. Few studies showed a significant association between apathy and disinhibition in patients with dementia [21] suggesting that apathy and disinhibition may alternate in the same persons. These individuals show disinhibited behaviors

Table 6B.2 Diagnostic criteria for apathy

1. Lack of motivation relative to patient's previous level of functioning or the standard of his/her age and culture
2. Presence, with lack of motivation, of at least one symptom belonging to each of the following three domains:
   Diminished goal-directed behavior: lack of affect, dependency on others to structure activity
   Diminished goal-directed cognition: lack of interest in learning new things or new experiences, lack of concern about one's personal problems
   Diminished concomitants of goal-directed behavior: unchanging affect, lack of emotional responsively to positive or negative events
3. The symptoms cause clinically significant distress or impairment in social, occupational, or other important areas of functioning
4. The symptoms are not due to a diminished level of consciousness or the direct physiological effects of a substance (such as a medication or drug abuse)

Marin [18].

sporadically, whilst apathy is present most of the time. A study of apathy in dementia showed that patients with apathy but no depression rarely report anhedonia, suggesting that anhedonia is more characteristic of depression than apathy.

Nakaaki *et al.* [22] explored the relationship between apathy/depression and executive function. They found that the deficits in executive function assessed by the Frontal Assessment Battery (FAB) and divided attention assessed by the dual task paradigm were larger in AD patients with both apathy and depression compared with patients with either apathy or depression alone. Patients with apathy have impaired ability to care for themselves and others; they show impaired role functioning; they are difficult to engage in treatment. A recent report [23] revealed that AD patients with apathy at baseline or those who developed apathy during follow-up had a significant increase in parkinsonism at follow-up when compared with patients with no apathy. Apathy may be an early manifestation of a more aggressive AD phenotype characterized by loss of motivation, increasing parkinsonism, and a faster cognitive and functional decline.

Quite a few instruments are currently used to measure the severity of apathy in dementia. The Apathy Evaluation Scale (AES) [24] is an 18-item scale which can be administered as a self-rated scale or as a clinician-operated test. Robert *et al.* [25] proposed the Apathy Inventory to separately assess apathy for emotional blunting, lack of initiative, and loss of interest. It was validated in AD, mild cognitive impairment (MCI), and Parkinson's disease. Recently, the Lille Apathy Rating Scale (LARS) [26] was developed and validated in Parkinson's disease. The NPI [7] is a multi-domain instrument to assess the caregiver's opinion on the patient. Apathy is one of these domains to evaluate.

Differential diagnosis of apathy includes abulia, despair, and the negative syndrome. *Abulia* is a state of loss, lack, or impairment of the power of the will to execute what is in mind in an individual without muscular problems. The eight features of abulia comprise (1) difficulty to initiate and sustain purposeful movements; (2) poverty of spontaneous movements; (3) reduced spontaneous speech; (4) increased response time to queries; (5) passivity; (6) reduced emotional responsiveness and spontaneity; (7) reduced social interaction; and (8) reduced interest in usual pastimes. *Despair* or *demoralization* is a psychological state occurring in normal individuals in response to the experience of overwhelming stress or significant changes in their personal and/or social environment. *The negative syndrome:* schizophrenia has two types of symptoms. The positive symptoms refer to an excess or distortion of normal functions (e.g., delusions or hallucinations). The negative symptoms represent a diminution or loss of normal functions (e.g., lack of spontaneous and flow of conversation, stereotyped thinking). The negative syndrome in schizophrenia is more complex than apathy in neurological diseases. Apathy is not related to either the positive symptoms or to depressive symptoms of schizophrenia, suggesting that apathy is an independent behavioral domain. It was reported to be the strongest predictor of poor functional outcome in schizophrenia.

Anxiety

An attempt to validate a set of DSM-IV constructs for generalized anxiety disorder (GAD) in dementia suggested excessive anxiety and worry as the key criterion and at least three of a list, including restlessness, irritability, muscle tension, excessive fears, and respiratory symptoms of anxiety, as additional criteria [27]. Anxiety in AD is a frequent comorbid condition of major depression. DeLuca and coworkers [28] found that elderly individuals with comorbid GAD and depression had a significantly greater decline in memory than depressed individuals without GAD. Porter *et al.* [29] reported that anxiety was more common in patients with VaD and frontotemporal dementia (FTD) than in patients with AD. In AD, anxiety was inversely related to Mini-Mental State Examination (MMSE) score (i.e., worse with more severe dementia), was more prevalent among patients with a younger age at onset (under age 65), and correlated with disability.

Agitation and aggression

Inappropriate behaviors [30] are divided into four main subtypes: (1) physically aggressive behaviors, such as hitting, kicking, or biting; (2) physically non-aggressive behaviors, such as pacing or inappropriately handling objects; (3) verbally non-aggressive agitation, such as constant repetition of sentences or requests; and (4) verbal aggression, such as cursing or screaming. Agitated behaviors can be assessed by the Cohen-Mansfield Agitation Inventory or as part of the subscale of the NPI or BEHAVE-AD. The Cohen-Mansfield Agitation Inventory is translated and validated in many Asian countries [31]. Agitation and aggression are frequently occurring and distressing behavioral symptoms in dementia. These symptoms cause risk to the patient and others, and confer a major management challenge for clinicians. Mild cognitive impairment patients frequently manifested neuropsychiatric symptoms. The most common symptoms in the MCI group [32] were dysphoria (39%), apathy (39%), irritability (29%), and anxiety (25%). There were significant differences in apathy, dysphoria, irritability, anxiety, agitation, and aberrant motor behavior between the MCI and control groups. Senanarong *et al.* [33] reported that there was no difference in agitation subscale scores of the NPI among patients with dementia of various etiologies. In patients with AD, there was increased prevalence of agitation with increasing dementia severity. Agitation contributed substantially to caregiver burden and impact. Delusion, disinhibition, and irritability subscale scores in AD patients were correlated with agitation across disease severity. Subscale scores of frontally mediated behaviors including irritability, delusions, and disinhibition predicted most of the variance in agitation levels. They concluded that frontal lobe dysfunction may predispose AD patients to agitation by exaggerating behavioral responses to many types of coexisting psychopathology or environmental provocations.

Disinhibition is a common behavioral disturbance in FTD and Parkinson's disease. It is found less commonly in AD. Disinhibition influences social behavior, resulting in excessive outgoingness, and violation of interpersonal norms. Starkstein *et al.* [34] demonstrated the phenomenology of disinhibition by performing factor analysis of the disinhibition scale scores in patients with AD. They found that the construct of disinhibition consists of four independent sub-syndromes: (1) abnormal motor behavior, (2) hypomania, (3) loss of insight and egocentrism, and (4) poor self-care. Disinhibition was significantly correlated with major and dysthymic depression, more severe negative symptoms, and loss of awareness. Most patients with disinhibition at the initial evaluation still showed disinhibition at follow-up indicating that disinhibition is a frequent and long-lasting problem in dementia. Senanarong *et al.* [35] conducted a study exploring a relationship among instrumental activities of daily living (IADL), agitation, apathy, and disinhibition in Thai AD patients. Instrumental activities of daily living depend on executive planning and procedural memory mediated by the frontal lobes. Neuropsychiatric symptoms are also mediated by frontal lobes. They found significant correlations between Thai IADL scores and agitation ($r = 0.350$), apathy ($r = 0.441$), and disinhibition ($r = 0.417$). After controlling for Thai Mental State Examination (TMSE), a significant correlation remained between Thai IADL scores and agitation ($r = 0.291$) and apathy ($r = 0.342$). These findings emphasize the important relationships between behavioral changes and impaired IADL.

Aberrant motor activity

Non-aggressive motor behavior such as inappropriate disrobing or constant questioning can cause annoyance among caregivers. Wandering and pacing become more problematic as the dementia severity progresses. Increased aberrant motor activity (AMA) in AD is associated with high neurofibrillary tangle loads in left orbitofrontal cortex [36]. This may reflect disinhibition drive on aberrant motor behaviors. However, a SPECT study [37] on AD with AMA showed hypoperfusion in the left parietotemporal areas. This may reflect problems in visuospatial attention causing AMA.

Psychosis

Psychotic symptoms such as hallucinations, delusions, and persistent misinterpretations are recognized comorbidities of dementia, especially AD. The prevalence of psychosis in AD is between 30% and 50% [38]. The occurrence of psychosis in dementia contributes to earlier institutionalization, accelerated cognitive deterioration, and increased caregiver burden. Delusions are unshakable false beliefs which are out of context with the person's social and cultural background. Hallucinations are false perceptions which are not just simply distortions or misinterpretations. The delusions in AD are often paranoid type, simple, and non-bizarre. Misidentification is common in AD. Content-specific delusions predominate in dementia [39]. Misidentification and reduplication syndromes with beliefs that places (called reduplicative paramnesia), people (called Capgras or Fregoli), or events are transformed in identity or duplication occur. Confabulation and anosognosia are related to delusions. Paranoid delusions involve that patient's spouse is having an affair (delusion of infidelity), or that someone steals patient's things (delusion of theft). Confabulation refers to incorrect statements made without conscious effort to deceive. It is associated with memory and executive dysfunction. Lee *et al.* reported that confabulations in remembering the past and planning the future are associated with delusions and aggression in AD [40,41]. The delusional AD produced more confabulations on episodic subjects than on semantic subjects. Visual hallucinations in persons with dementia are often complex and well-formed. Auditory hallucinations commonly involve hearing voices of diseased persons or of those who are not in the room. Psychosis in AD is a distinct syndrome markedly different from schizophrenia in older persons (Table 6B.3). New criteria of psychosis in AD [38] and other dementia will exclude psychosis secondary to delirium, other generalized medical conditions, substance use, and primary psychotic disorders. The psychosis in AD is often accompanied with agitation, negative symptoms, and depression.

Behavioral features of major dementia and MCI

Alzheimer's disease features an array of neuropsychiatric symptoms including apathy, agitation, depression, anxiety. Occurrence of agitation and psychosis in AD is commonly found in severe stages. The European Alzheimer Disease Consortium performed factor analysis of NPI on over 2000 AD patients to identify subsyndromes [42] of the NPI. They discovered four neuropsychiatric subsyndromes: hyperactivity, psychosis, affective symptoms, and apathy. These four factors explained 51.8% of the total variance in the data. Hyperactivity had high loadings on agitation, disinhibition, irritability, and AMA. Psychosis dimension includes delusions, hallucinations, and nighttime behavior disturbances. An affective dimension had high loading on depression and anxiety. Apathy dimension had high loading on apathy and appetite and eating abnormality. The most common subsyndrome was the apathy (65%), followed by the hyperactivity (64%), affective (59%), and psychosis (38%).

Vascular dementia(VaD) in Asia

Fuh *et al.* [9] demonstrated that cortical VaD had the highest mean composite NPI score in all domains, while AD patients had the lowest composite NPI score in most domains. The mean composite score of the apathy and sleep

Table 6B.3 Comparison of psychosis in Alzheimer's disease with schizophrenia in older persons

	Psychosis in AD	*Schizophrenia*
Frequency	30–50% of people with dementia	<1% of general population
Complex delusions	Rare	Frequent
Misidentification of caregivers	Frequent	Rare
Common form of hallucinations	Visual	Auditory
Schneider first-rank symptoms	Rare	Frequent
Suicidal ideation	Rare	Frequent
Past history of psychosis	Rare	Very common
Remission of psychosis	Frequent	Uncommon
Maintenance of antipsychotics	Less than a year	Need many years
Average daily dose of antipsychotics	15–25% of young adults with schizophrenia	40–60% of young adults with schizophrenia

Jests and Finkel [38].

disturbance domains in patients with cortical VaD were significantly higher than those in AD. Chiu and coworkers [43] studied 157 participants with vascular cognitive impairment (VCI), 41 had vascular cognitive impairment non-dementia (CIND), 95 had VaD, 21 had mixed AD and VaD. Sleep disturbance was the most common symptom in all patient groups. Apathy is significantly lower in vascular CIND compared with mixed AD and VaD. Patients with VaD had the highest mean composite NPI scores in most domains and vascular CIND patients had the lowest composite scores in most domains. Behavioral disturbances frequently arise from cerebrovascular disease regardless of the development of dementia. (See also Chapters 4A and 4B.)

Parkinson's disease dementia (PDD)

Aarsland *et al.* [44] reported on 537 patients with PDD. Eighty-nine percent of the patients presented at least one symptom on the NPI, 77% had two or more symptoms and 64% had at least one symptom with a score > or = 4. The most common symptoms were depression (58%), apathy (54%), anxiety (49%), and hallucinations (44%). Patients with more severe dementia and advanced Parkinson's disease had more neuropsychiatric symptoms. Five NPI clusters were identified: one group with few and mild symptoms; a mood cluster; apathy; agitation; and a psychosis cluster. The psychosis and agitation clusters had the lowest MMSE score and the highest Unified

Table 6B.4 Neuropsychiatric and behavioral features of major dementia

Dementia type	*Common neuropsychiatric and behavioral features*
Mild cognitive impairment (amnestic type)	Depression, apathy, anxiety, irritability
Alzheimer's disease	Apathy, agitation, depression, anxiety, irritability; delusions and hallucinations are found more frequently in severe stage
Vascular dementia	Apathy, depression, delusions
Dementia with Lewy bodies	Visual hallucinations, delusions, depression, rapid eye movement (REM) sleep behavioral disorder
Parkinson's disease dementia	Visual hallucinations, delusions, depression, rapid eye movement (REM) sleep behavioral disorder
Frontotemporal dementia	Apathy, disinhibition, euphoria, repetitive behaviors, eating changes
Progressive supranuclear palsy	Apathy, disinhibition
Corticobasal degeneration	Depression
Huntington's disease dementia	Dysphoria, agitation, irritability, apathy, anxiety

McKeith and Cummings [47], Pausen *et al.* [48], Shin *et al.* [49].

Parkinson's Disease Rating Scale and caregiver distress scores.

Frontotemporal dementia (FTD)

Bozeat and coworkers [45] examined 33 patients with (FTD), comprising 20 with temporal variant FTD (tv FTD) or semantic dementia and 13 with frontal variant FTD (fv FTD). Factor analysis showed four meaningful symptom clusters: (1) stereotypic and altered eating behavior; (2) executive dysfunction and self-care; (3) mood changes; and (4) loss of social awareness. Only stereotypic and altered eating behavior and loss of social awareness reliably differentiated AD from FTD with no effect of disease severity. The patients with fv FTD and semantic dementia were behaviorally similar, reflecting the involvement of a common network, the ventral frontal lobe, temporal pole, and amygdala.

Mild cognitive impairment (MCI)

A recent review on neuropsychiatric manifestations of MCI [46] revealed that behavioral disturbances are found in 35–75% of MCI patients. Most common neuropsychiatric symptoms are depression, apathy, anxiety, and irritability. The behavioral changes observed in MCI are similar to those in AD. Table 6B.4 outlines the neuropsychiatric and behavioral features of major dementia. Mild cognitive impairment patients with behavioral features are more prone to develop AD than those without neuropsychiatric problems.

Conclusion

Etiological factors that underlie neuropsychiatric and behavioral problems in patients with dementia are multifaceted, and are influenced to a great deal by biological and non-biological antecedents. There is an emerging literature that describes well, and classifies, the behavioral and psychological symptoms of dementia (BPSD), resulting in neuropsychiatric subsyndromes of dementia. While, hitherto, the vast majority of research has been confined to the West, there are now emerging data from Asian and other non-western cultures enabling greater understanding of transcultural factors. The management of dementia should ideally address these specific subsyndromes while taking into account the transcultural factors that will no doubt impact on outcome.

References

1. Cummings JL. Neuropsychiatric and behavioral alterations and their management in moderate to severe Alzheimer's disease. *Neurology* 2005; **65**: S18–24.
2. Chow TW, Liu CK, Fuh JL, Leung VP, Tai CT, Chen LW, *et al.* Neuropsychiatric symptoms of Alzheimer's disease differ in Chinese and American patients. *Int J Geriatr Psychiatry* 2002; **17**: 22–8.
3. Chiu MJ, Chen TF, Yip PK, Hua MS, Tang LY. Behavioral and psychologic symptoms in different types of dementia. *J Formos Med Assoc* 2006; **105** (7): 556–62.
4. Finklel SI, Burns A, Cohen G. Behavioral and psychological symptoms of dementia (BPSD): a clinical and research update, overview. *Int Psychogeriatr* 2000; **12**: 13–18.
5. Mack JL, Patterson MB, Tariot PN. Behavior Rating Scale for Dementia: development of test scales and presentation of data for 555 individuals with Alzheimer's Disease. *J Geriatr Psychiatry Neurol* 1999; **12**: 211–23.
6. Reisberg B, Borenstein J, Salob SP, *et al.* Behavioral symptoms in Alzheimer's disease: phenomenology and treatment. *J Clin Psychiatry* 1987; **48**(Suppl): 9–15.
7. Cummings JL. The Neuropsychiatric Inventory: assessing psychopathology in dementia patients. *Neurology* 1997; **48**(Suppl 6): S10–16.
8. Suh GH, Kim SK. Behavioral and psychological signs and symptoms of dementia (BPSD) in antipsychotic-naïve Alzheimer's disease patients. *Int Psychogeriatr* 2004; **16**: 337–50.
9. Fuh JL, Wang SJ, Cummings JL. Neuropsychiatric profiles in patients with Alzheimer's disease and vascular dementia. *J Neurol Neurosurg Psychiatry* 2005; **76**: 1337–41.
10. Sink KM, Holden KF, Yaffy K. Pharmacological treatment of neuropsychiatric symptoms of dementia: a review of the evidence. *JAMA* 2005; **293**: 596–608.
11. Olin JT, Schneider LS, Katz IR, *et al.* Provisional diagnostic criteria for depression of Alzheimer disease. *Am J Psychiatry* 2002; **10**: 125–8.
12. American Psychiatric Association *Diagnostic and Statistical Manual of Mental Disorders*, 4th edn. Washington, DC, American Psychiatric Association, 1994.
13. Teng E, Ringman JM, Ross LK, *et al.* Diagnosing depression in Alzheimer disease with the National Institute of Mental Health provisional criteria. *Am J Psychiatry* 2008; **16**: 469–77.
14. Starkstein SE, Jorge R, Mizrahi R, Robinson RG. The construct of minor and major depression in

Alzheimer's disease. *Am J Psychiatry* 2005; **162**: 2086–93.

15. Mayer LS, Bay RC, Politis A, *et al.* Comparison of three rating scales as outcome measures for treatment trials of depression in Alzheimer disease: findings from DIADS. *Int J Geriatr Psychiatry* 2006; **21**: 930–6.
16. Pang FC, Chow TW, Cummings JL, *et al.* Effect of neuropsychiatric symptoms of Alzheimer's disease on Chinese and American caregivers. *Int J Geriatr Psychiatry* 2002; **17**: 29–34.
17. Starkstein SE, Petracca G, Chemerinski E, Kremer J. Syndromic validity of apathy in Alzheimer's disease. *Am J Psychiatry* 2001; **158**: 872–7.
18. Marin RS. Apathy: a neuropsychiatric syndrome. *J Neuropsychiatry Clin Neurosci* 1991; **3**: 243–54.
19. Levy R, Dubois B. Apathy and functional anatomy of the prefrontal cortex-basal ganglia circuits. *Cereb Cortex* 2006; **16**: 916–28.
20. Fuh JL, Lam L, Hirono N, Senanarong V, Cummings JL. Neuropsychiatric inventory workshop: behavioral and psychologic symptoms of dementia in Asia. *Alzheimer Dis Assoc Disord* 2006; **20**: 314–17.
21. Starkstein SE, Garau ML, Cao A. Prevalence and clinical correlates of disinhibition in dementia. *Cogn Behav Neurol* 2004; **17**: 139–47.
22. Nakaaki S, Murata Y, Sato J, *et al.* Association between apathy/depression and executive function in patients with Alzheimer's disease. *Int Psychogeriatr* 2008; **20**: 964–75.
23. Starkstein SE, Merello M, Brockman S, *et al.* Apathy predicts more severe Parkinsonism in Alzheimer's disease. *Am J Geriatr Psychiatry* 2009; **17**: 1–8.
24. Marin RS, Biedrycki RC, Firiciogullari S. Reliability and validity of the Apathy Evaluation Scale. *Psychiatry Res* 1991; **38**(2): 143–62.
25. Robert PH, Clairet S, Benoit M, *et al.* The apathy inventory assessment of apathy and awareness in Alzheimer's disease, Parkinson's disease and mild cognitive impairment. *Int J Geriatr Psychiatry* 2002; **17**: 1099–105.
26. Sockeel P, Dujardin K, Devos D, *et al.* The Lille apathy rating scale (LARS), a new instrument for detecting and quantifying apathy: validation in Parkinson's disease. *J Neurol Neurosurg Psychiatry* 2006; **777**: 579–84.
27. Starkstein SE, Jorge R, Petracca G, Robinson R. The construct of generalized anxiety disorder in Alzheimer disease. *Am J Geriatr Psychiatry* 2007; **15**: 42–9.
28. DeLuca AK, Lenze EJ, Mulsant BH, *et al.* Comorbid anxiety disorder in late life depression: association with memory decline over four years. *Int J Geriatr Psychiatry* 2005; **20**: 848–54.
29. Porter VR, Buxton WG, Fairbanks LA, *et al.* Frequency and characteristics of anxiety among patients with Alzheimer's disease and related dementias. *J Neuropsychiatry Clin Neurosci* 2003; **15**: 180–6.
30. Cohen-Mansfield J, Werner P, Watson V, *et al.* Agitation among elderly persons at adult day-care centers: the experiences of relatives and staff members. *Int Psychogeriatr* 1995; 7: 447–58.
31. Suh GH. Agitation behaviors among the institutionsalized elderly with dementia: validation of the Korean version of the Cohen-Mansfield Agitation Inventory. *Int J Geriatr Psychiatry* 2004; **19**: 378–85.
32. Hwang TJ, Masterman DL, Ortiz R, Fairbanks LA, Cummings JL. Mild cognitive impairment is associated with characteristic neuropsychiatric symptoms. *Alzheimer Dis Assoc Disord* 2004; **18**: 17–21.

33. Senanarong V, Cummings JL, Fairbanks L, *et al.* Agitation in Alzheimer's disease is a manifestation of frontal lobe dysfunction. *Dement Geriatr Cogn Disord* 2004; **17**: 14–20.

34. Starkstein SE, Garau ML, Cao A. Prevalence and clinical correlates of disinhibition in dementia. *Cogn Behav Neurol* 2004; **17**: 139–47.

35. Senanarong V, Poungvarin N, Jamjumras P, *et al.* Neuropsychiatric symptoms, functional impairment and executive ability in Thai patients with Alzheimer's disease. *Int Psychogeriatr* 2005; **17**: 81–90.

36. Tekin S, Mega MS, Masterman DM, *et al.* Orbitofrontal and anterior cingulated cortex neurofibrillary tangle burden is associated with agitation in Alzheimer's disease. *Ann Neurol* 2001; **49**: 355–61.

37. Rolland Y, Payoux P, Lauwers-Cances V *et al.* A SPECT study of wandering behavior in Alzheimer's disease. *Int J Geriatr Psychiatry* 2005; **20**: 816–20.

38. Jests DV, Finkel SI. Psychosis of Alzheimer's disease and related dementias. Diagnostic criteria for a distinct syndrome. *Am J Geriatr Psychiatry* 2000; **8**: 29–34.

39. Devinsky O. Delusional misidentifications and duplications. Right brain lesions, left brain delusions. *Neurology* 2009; **72**: 80–7.

40. Lee E, Akanuma K, Meguro M, *et al.* Confabulations in remembering past and planning future are associated with psychiatric symptoms in Alzheimer's disease. *Arch Clin Neuropsychol* 2007; **22**: 949–56.

41. Lee E, Meguro K, Hashimoto R, *et al.* Confabulations in episodic memory are associated with delusions in Alzheimer's disease. *J Geriatr Psychiatry Neurol* 2007; **20**: 34–40.

42. Alten P, Verhey FR, Bozik M, *et al.* Neuropsychiatric syndromes in dementia. Results from the European Alzheimer Disease Consortium: Part I. *Dement Geriatr Cogn Disord* 2007; **24**: 457–63.

43. Chiu PJ, Liu CH, Tsai CH. Neuropsychiatric manifestations in vascular cognitive impairment patients with and without dementia. *Acta Neurol Taiwan* 2007; **16**: 86–91.

44. Aarsland D, Brønnick K, Ehrt U, *et al.* Neuropsychiatric symptoms in patients with Parkinson's disease and dementia: frequency, profile and associated care giver stress. *J Neurol Neurosurg Psychiatry* 2007; **78**: 36–42.

45. Bozeat S, Gregory CA, Ralph MAL, Hodges JR. Which neuropsychiatric and behavioral features distinguish frontal and temporal variants of frontotemporal dementia from Alzheimer's Disease? *J Neurol Neurosurg Psychiatry* 2000; **69**: 178–86.

46. Apostolova LG, Cummings JL. Neuropsychiatric manifestations in mild cognitive impairment: a systematic review of the literature. *Dement Geriatr Cogn Disord* 2008; **25**: 115–26.

47. McKeith I, Cummings JL. Behavioral changes and psychological symptoms in dementia disorders. *Lancet Neurol* 2005; **4**: 735–42.

48. Pausen JS, Ready RE, Hamilton JM, Mega MS, Cummings JL. Neuropsychiatric aspects of Huntington's disease. *J Neurol Neurosurg Psychiatry* 2001; **71**: 310–14.

49. Shin IS, Carter M, Masterman D, Fairbanks L, Cummings JL. Neuropsychiatric symptoms and quality of life in Alzheimer's disease. *Am J Geriatr Psychiatry* 2005; **13**: 469–74.

Psychosocial factors

Quality of life in dementia: global perspective and transcultural issues

Caroline Selai, Demetris Pillas, and Annabel Dodds

Introduction

The measurement of health-related quality of life (HR-QoL) raises many methodological issues. These issues become more complex when assessing HR-QoL of a person with dementia, especially if HR-QoL is being compared across cultures. The operational definition and assessment of HR-QoL must take into account the local culture and value systems. Researchers need to be aware of the methodological issues, including protocols for the multiple steps of translation of tools, ensuring conceptual equivalence, the stages of psychometric testing, and grounding of assessments in the traditional concepts of health in each culture.

This chapter highlights some of the key debates and research studies from the large and growing literature.

Assessment of quality of life

Definition

Although the definition of this somewhat elusive term is still occasionally discussed in the literature, there is general consensus on some fundamental points. First, although the phrases "quality of life," "health-related quality of life," and "health status" are used somewhat interchangeably, there is broad agreement that, in the medical context, QoL should be regarded as a *multidimensional* construct comprising: physical, psychological, and social well-being [1]. Second, since appraisal of QoL is highly subjective, any appraisal of QoL should rely, where possible, on the perception of the individual patient.

Why assess quality of life?

Whilst QoL measures have been developed for a number of reasons [2] (see Table 7A.1), two basic aspects of health care underlie most of the questions that QoL appraisals set out to answer: outcome of treatment and cost. With increasingly sophisticated life-saving and life-prolonging medical interventions, QoL has emerged as an important outcome. Also, it is

Dementia: A Global Approach, ed. Ennapadam S. Krishnamoorthy, Martin J. Prince, and Jeffrey L. Cummings. Published by Cambridge University Press.

Table 7A.1 Applications of quality-of-life measures

- Screening and monitoring for psychosocial problems in individual patient care
- Population surveys of perceived health problems
- Medical audit
- Outcome measures in health services or evaluation research
- Clinical trials
- Cost–utility analyses

From Fitzpatrick *et al.* [3].

argued that no country in the world can *afford* to do all that it is technically possible to do to improve the health of its citizens and so the need has arisen for some system of setting priorities.

Types of QoL measures

There is no "gold standard" for measuring QoL and there is a wide range of instruments available, or in development. In brief, *generic* instruments cover a broad range of QoL domains in a single instrument. Their chief advantage is in facilitating comparisons among different disease groups. *Disease-specific* instruments reduce patient burden by including only relevant items for a particular illness but their main disadvantage is the lack of comparability of results with those from other disease groups. *Health profiles* provide separate scores for each of the dimensions of QoL, whereas a *health index,* a type of generic instrument, gives a single summary score, usually from 0 (death) to 1 (perfect health). A further category, developed within the economic tradition, is that of *utility* measures, which are based on preferences for health states. Where the focus is on *society* as a whole and the societal allocation of scarce resources, such preference-weighted measures are required. The choice of measure will depend upon the goal of the study.

QoL in dementia: conceptual issues

A number of conceptual issues need to be considered in the measurement of QoL in dementia. Assessment of well-being in any patient is complex. The process becomes even more difficult if the patient has a degenerating, dementing condition.

Cognitive function

Lezak [4] postulates four major classes of cognitive functions and it can be seen that self-appraisal of QoL or well-being involves each one of these:

1. *receptive functions:* abilities to select, acquire, classify, and integrate information;
2. *memory and learning:* information storage and retrieval;
3. *thinking:* mental organization and reorganization of information;
4. *expressive functions:* means through which information is communicated or acted upon.

Whilst many disorders such as Alzheimer's disease come under the heading *dementias*, dementia is commonly defined as *global cognitive decline* [4].

Quality-of-life assessment comprises a highly complex procedure of introspection and evaluation, involving several components of cognition including implicit and explicit memory [2]. Patient's self-ratings will be influenced by education, memory, and attention difficulties [5]. If the patient is no longer able to appraise their own QoL, researchers may consider obtaining proxy reports.

Loss of insight

Loss of insight has been thought to be part of the general cognitive collapse in dementia [6]. Strong associations have been found between awareness of memory deficit and disturbed mood, particularly depression and irritability, in patients with Alzheimer's disease (AD) [7]. Depression is a common comorbidity of dementia [8] and mood disturbances may have an important impact on QOL.

Anosognosia

Patients with dementia may be unaware of their deficit; they may have anosognosia [9]. At interview the patient will often describe him/herself as "well" and even on probing will admit to no problems.

Neuropsychiatric symptoms

Neuropsychiatric disturbances are common manifestations of dementing disorders [10]. Patients with AD experience delusions, agitation, anxiety, and personality changes, and neuropsychiatric disorders may be the presenting manifestations of the disease [11] (see Chapter 6B on behavioral and psychological symptoms of dementia).

Stages of dementia

Any appraisal of QoL in dementia must take account of the different stages of dementia, the degree of insight, and variation in aspects of neuropsychological decline. Account will need to be taken of whether the patient can function independently, of whether he/she can live alone, and of comorbidity.

Proxy reports

Proxy reports have been reviewed [12,13]. Studies of proxy-derived data suggest that: (1) the more objective the question and the more concrete the item in question, the closer the proxy's response will be to the subject's; (2) proxies are poorer reporters for conditions and symptoms that are private and not easily observed; (3) findings regarding proxy-subject agreement for ratings of affective status are inconsistent.

Perhaps the most consistent findings across studies are that greater agreement is obtained for objective items that ask about discrete, observable aspects of functioning such as mobility, and that proxies tend to over-rate disability, compared to patients' own reports.

Review of key QoL instruments in dementia

The development of instruments and the choice of a tool depend on the goal of the study. A number of QoL assessment techniques are in development and full testing of their psychometric properties is ongoing.

The Schedule for the Evaluation of Individual Quality of Life (SEIQoL)

Patients with dementia are asked to rate their own QoL using the individualized measure, the SEIQOL. With this approach, devised from a technique known as judgment analysis, patients rate their level of functioning in five self-nominated facets of life and then indicate the relative weight or importance they attach to each [14].

The Quality of Life-AD (QoL-AD)

The Quality of Life-AD (QoL-AD) obtains a rating of the patient's QoL from both the patient and the caregiver [15]. The scale is based on a literature review on QoL in older adults and on the assessment of QoL in other chronically ill populations. It comprises 13 items covering the domains of physical health, energy, mood, living situation, memory, family, marriage, friends, chores, fun, money, self, and life as a whole.

Dementia QoL (DQoL)

This instrument has been designed for direct respondent assessment in cognitively impaired populations [16]. The DQoL has five domains: self-esteem; positive affect/humor; negative affect; feelings of belonging; and sense of aesthetics, with a total of 29 items. Psychometric testing has shown this to be a reliable and valid instrument [16].

The Community Dementia QoL Profile (CDQLP)

This is a disease-specific, self-administered instrument which consists of two sections. Part I is a measure of the patient's QoL assessed by his/her carer as a proxy and part II is a measure of the carer's own QoL and stress [17].

The ADRQL (Alzheimer's Disease-Related Quality of Life) Instrument

The ADRQL (Alzheimer's Disease-Related Quality of Life) is a multidimensional, disease-specific, health-related QoL instrument, developed for use in evaluations of treatment interventions in AD [18]. It has five domains: social interaction; awareness of self; feelings and mood; enjoyment of activities; and response to surroundings. The instrument is proxy-rated.

Cognitively Impaired Life Quality Scale (CILQ)

This instrument measures the QoL of profoundly impaired patients through nursing caregivers' eyes [19]. A 29-item version of the CILQ and a shortened, 14-item version of the scale are being developed.

Quality of Life Assessment Schedule (QoLAS)

The QoLAS is a semi-structured interview technique for assessing QoL. At interview, the respondent is invited to recount what is important for his/her QoL and ways in which their current health condition is affecting their QoL. Key constructs are extracted from this narrative. In total, ten "constructs" are elicited, two for each of the following domains of QoL: physical, psychological, social/family, daily activities, and cognitive functioning (or well-being). The respondent is next asked to rate how much of a problem each of these is now on a 0–5 scale.

Dementia-specific cross-cultural issues

Cross-cultural research: methodological issues

The importance of cultural influences on QoL is reflected in the World Health Organization (WHO) definition of QoL as "the perception of individuals of their own position in life in the context of the culture and value systems in which they live." [20].

In cross-cultural QoL research there are, broadly, two schools of thought: some think that issues of relevance to health or QoL are similar across cultures and that the careful translation of instruments is all that is important. The second school, influenced by sociologists and anthropologists, is that perceptions of QoL are "culture bound." It is argued that to assess QoL in a culturally sensitive way, researchers must study the beliefs and behaviors in the context of the culture to which they belong [21]. Therefore, translations of instruments developed in Western cultures may not be valid in other societies. Guidelines, based on these considerations, have been developed for culturally sensitive research, both in terms of the development and translation of questionnaires and cross-cultural study design [22].

If one accepts the translatability of QoL instruments, the first stage is forward-translation of the original questionnaire into the target language. It is important that not only the literal meaning of the words is translated but that the meaning of the question does not change. The aim is to reach conceptual equivalence rather than purely terminological equivalence. The second stage is back-translation. The translation reports are independently reviewed. The aim is to preserve the original meaning of the questionnaire, rather than emphasis on the best "literal" translation. Second, the psychometric properties (validity, reliability, and responsiveness) need to be tested in the target culture. A third issue is to assess whether there is any difference in the pattern of acceptance and response to questionnaires in the particular cultures. For example, people in some cultures may not be familiar with completing questionnaires, they may see them as intrusive, or there may be a high level of illiteracy. Thus, QoL measures need to be based on the traditional concepts of health in each culture, in order to have face validity in that culture.

Key issues in dementia-specific transcultural research

1. Definition of dementia: operationally defined in the same way across cultures?
2. Diagnosis of dementia: (a) time and manner of presentation to health professionals, (b) appropriateness of measures standardized and validated in one culture for use in another?
3. Validity of neuropsychological testing, e.g., Mini-Mental State Examination (MMSE),

National Adult Reading Test (NART) in cultures with low literacy.
4. Do all cultures recognize cognitive decline as a "major problem that needs tackling" or are these changes seen as part of normal behavior?
5. Attitudes of family members – assessment of burden of caring in developing countries, and attitudes to institutionalization.
6. Cost of care and cost of research in developing countries.

Transcultural QoL research in dementia: summary of key themes

Research on the transcultural aspects of dementia research is growing and mainly focuses on four key areas: (1) cultural attitudes to aging, cognitive decline, and variations in the presentation of dementia; (2) epidemiological studies; (3) differences in care and the services offered to people with dementia; and (4) the use of psychometric scales and screening instruments across cultures.

Attitudes to aging, decline in cognitive capacities, and dementia

Attitudes to dementia differ according to culture. For example, many people accept even a significant decline in cognitive abilities and health status as a normal part of aging. In a study of QoL from the view point of patients with dementia in Japan, where dementia is just another stage in life, to be embraced and accepted, QoL was defined by criteria such as happiness and spiritual abundance. After confrontation and acceptance, the patients in this survey showed more positive attitudes and behavior, e.g., dancing and singing spontaneously [23].

A study of accounts given by family and health professionals caring for people with dementia in South Korea showed that young Koreans, who believe in Confucian values such as filial piety and duty to care for elders, expect elders to become dependent as they age [24]. They strive to maintain family harmony, rejecting nursing care. Those carers that see dementia as "normal" do not seek help and neither do those who see it as a form of mental illness (for fear or stigmatization). The carer is almost always a daughter-in-law, otherwise a daughter or, very rarely, a son. There is no meaningful state support. Attitudes are changing amongst the younger generation, who are moving away from Confucian values, and amongst the middle-aged who don't want to create such a burden for their children (see also Chapters 9B, 9E, and 9F on caregiving from Africa, Japan, and China).

In a study of attitudes to dementia amongst four ethnic groups (African Americans, Asian Americans, Latinos, and Anglo European Americans), three models of understanding were found: biomedical, mixed biomedical and folk, folk [25]. A total of 36% used the biomedical model only, 54% used mixed biomedical and folk, and only 10% used folk only (i.e., stress, aging, confusion, craziness, mental illness, tough life.) This was just a convenience sample and therefore the results may not be generalizable to the general population of dementia caregivers.

In a study of African American (n = 5) and White (n = 5) caregivers of persons with AD and related disorders [26], all responded that their ethnicity influenced how they cared for their charges, as did spirituality and religion.

It seems that both black and white people turn to "God" in times of emotional need, which would suggest a complex interaction between ethnicity and religious practice. Again, the sample size was small.

Cultural differences in acceptance of cognitive decline (and presentation to healthcare providers) may explain apparent differences in prevalence of dementia. In a study of four ethnic groups in Singapore, vascular dementia was found to be more prevalent than AD, especially amongst Chinese and Malays, whereas AD was more prevalent than vascular dementia amongst Indians and Eurasians [27]. Malays were underrepresented in this study but have highest prevalence of dementia out of the three ethnic groups and one explanation is that acceptance of cognitive decline is poor in this group. There is selection bias because this was a clinical (not a community) study and those seeking medical attention might not have been representative of the community as a whole. Malays would have been underrepresented because they avoid health care and fewer would have been admitted to the dementia clinics studied.

Epidemiological studies

A key paper is the consensus statement from the "10/66 Dementia Research Group" [28]. This paper reports an important meeting which took place in Cochin, India, in 1999 to address the topic of dementia in developing countries. The focus was that only 10% of dementia research is directed at the 66% of people with dementia who actually live in developing countries. By 2020 this proportion will have risen to 75%. Research activity has been slow to reflect this radical change in demographics. It was also discussed that relatively little is known about the care arrangements of those older people who are affected. Discussion included the key research questions and how these should be prioritized. Recommendations made included greater collaboration between developed and developing countries, and the sharing of funds and expertise, thus giving "developing world" researchers the ability to plan their own local research which will be more culturally appropriate than a "Western" team going in and conducting research in a potentially less appropriate fashion.

An important study [29] addressed the problems of developing culturally and educationally sensitive screening tools for dementia. False positives attributable to depression and to people with low education in non-literate populations not performing well in tasks that require literacy skills are some problems encountered in these studies. The aim of this study was to develop and test a culturally and educationally unbiased diagnostic instrument for dementia.

In a multicenter study, the 10/66 Dementia Research Group interviewed 2885 people aged 60 years and older in 25 centers, most in universities, in India, China and South East Asia, Latin America and the Caribbean and Africa. It was found that putting together three screening tools for dementia diagnosis leads to a greater sensitivity than any of the screening tools alone.

In a study conducted in rural southern India, the prevalence of dementia was found to be 3.5% [30] with higher prevalence among lower socioeconomic classes (4.0%) than higher classes (1.8%). Each elderly person was given the Geriatric Mental State Schedule

(GMS) translated into Tamil, already standardized to the Indian population. Two psychiatrists performed clinical examinations using the International Classification of Diseases, tenth edition (ICD-10)[31] diagnostic criteria, blind to the GMS diagnosis. The inter-rater reliability of the psychiatrists was kappa 0.85, which is good. There was 100% response rate for the study, eliminating population bias. A number of difficulties were encountered, e.g., age was difficult to ascertain as the group was largely illiterate with an absence of birth registers. The events calendar technique was used to ascertain a reasonable approximation of age, along with personal events like year of attaining menarche, year of birth of first child, and historical events.

In an editorial, Rait and Burns [32] argue that in order to understand the illnesses, including mental illnesses amongst the South Asian community in the UK, which is large and diverse, comprising India, Pakistan, and Bangladesh, it is important to appreciate the background, culture, and context in order to recognize the "effects of their culture, experiences and environment." Learning about the attitudes that the elderly have towards mental illness, their "expressions of distress," "views on management and treatment," and use of health services will facilitate the introduction of appropriate healthcare protocols for the elderly of these ethnicities.

South Asian elderly face some problems common to all elderly people and some specific to themselves, such as discrimination in various areas of life from housing to employment [32].

It is argued that appropriate questioning may be the key to understanding what South Asians *really* think about mental health issues. This will include translation and interpretation of the sense of what is being said, not just direct literal translation which may miss delicate nuances conveying more subtle allusions to psychological illness worries.

An epidemiological study from Brazil found that the older population, and the number of people in their "third age," is growing rapidly, creating a pressing need for policies to deal with the social consequences, economic issues, and health provision for the aging population [33]. The elderly represent about 10% of the population, mostly women, widows, those with low education and with lower earnings than their male counterparts. Many of the people that care for elderly with dementia are themselves elderly and tend to develop psychiatric symptoms which can contribute to the demand for the already scarce mental health services.

Differences in care and service offered

A study of dementia care in England compared the social model of disability with the medical model, neither of which comprehensively capture the full range of issues [34]. Younger people with dementia (aged 65 or less) fall between care policies and sometimes lack appropriate care because of this. People with dementia from ethnic minority groups also fall through the net because they do not fulfil eligibility criteria for what is available. Neither group gets the most appropriate care.

In a study comparing the characteristics of clients and services provided for people with dementia in Sweden and the USA, several differences emerged in (1) admission criteria: the service providers in the USA usually don't admit patients with incontinence or disruptive behavior whereas in Sweden there are no restrictions on type of patients, with the exception of one or two day centers; (2) facilities: the USA has more specialist facilities, e.g., foot doctor, ophthalmologist, more family support services, e.g., counseling, case management whereas Sweden has fewer specialists, and no family support groups or dementia education for families; (3) activities: the USA offers more exercise, reminiscence activity, cognitive and music activity whereas in Sweden, activities are worked into daily life without being "formal" [35].

A study of African American caregivers, explored the reasons for the delays in getting people from this minority group evaluated [36]. Delays in sending patients for evaluation were partly a result of the tradition of respecting and protecting elders (see Chapter 9B from Nigeria) and partly attributable to deficit in knowledge about dementia. There is also a legacy of distrust amongst African Americans of the healthcare system and institutions. It is suggested that there is a need for cross-cultural training for healthcare providers.

In a study of ethnicity and time to institutionalization of dementia patients which compared Latina and Caucasian female family caregivers, it was found that Latinas delayed institutionalization significantly longer than their Caucasian counterparts. This could not be accounted for by care-recipient characteristics or caregiver demographics [37].

Psychometric scales and screening instruments

Even though a rating scale may have undergone extensive psychometric testing, it is important to fully validate the scale for use in another culture. QoL scales need to be properly translated according to international guidelines, ensuring they are grounded in the traditional concepts of health in each culture, and aiming to reach conceptual equivalence rather than purely terminological equivalence. The psychometric properties of any scale must be retested before use in another culture.

In order to identify those that are demented in an illiterate population group in North India, Ganguli *et al.* produced a Hindi adaptation of the MMSE [38]. This adaptation was useful to test the prevalence of dementia in both illiterate and literate populations. The Hindi adaptation of the MMSE had substitute sections so that the persons with no knowledge of reading/time etc. could be compared at a standardized level to those with an education. Modifications were made to "tap the same cognitive domains" in those that are not educated. Subtraction of serial sevens was the most difficult task for all groups and naming the watch was the easiest for all groups.

Similar issues arose on a paper using the Tamil GMS in a rural setting in India [39]. The study also pointed out the effect that low educational status can have on borderline "dementia" status as suggested by the GMS. This is a well-known concept as many of the tasks required to be tested in assessing dementia status involve literacy skills that the uneducated may never have acquired. The study concluded that AD, multi-infarct dementia and other dementias do exist in rural settings and pose a significant healthcare burden, at a prevalence of approximately 3.5%. More culturally fair measurements may give more accurate absolute numbers of people with dementia in rural India.

Conclusion

Researchers need to be aware of the methodological issues inherent in cross-cultural research including issues of translation, conceptual equivalence, psychometric testing, and grounding of assessments in the traditional concepts of health in each culture.

Research on the transcultural aspects of dementia is growing. Topics have included: cultural attitudes to aging, decline in cognitive capacities and dementia, and variations in the presentation of dementia; epidemiological studies; differences in care and the services offered to people with dementia; and the use of psychometric scales and screening instruments across cultures. This field of research is likely to grow significantly in the future.

References

1. Bowling A. *Measuring Disease: A Review of Disease-Specific Quality of Life Measurement Scales*. Buckingham, Open University Press, 1995.
2. Barofsky, I. Cognitive aspects of quality of life assessment. In: Spilker B, ed. *Quality of Life and Pharmacoeconomics in Clinical Trials*, 2nd edn. Philadelphia, Lippincott-Raven. 1996; 107–15.
3. Fitzpatrick R, Fletcher AE, Gore SM, *et al.* Quality of life measures in health care. I: Applications and issues in assessment. *BMJ* 1992; **305**: 1074–7.
4. Lezak MD. *Neuropsychological Assessment*, 3rd edn. New York, Oxford University Press, 1995.
5. Stewart AL, Sherbourne CD, Brod M. Measuring health-related quality of life in older and demented populations. In: Spilker B, ed. *Quality of Life and Pharmacoeconomics in Clinical Trials*, 2nd edn. Philadelphia, Lippincott-Raven. 1996; 819–30.
6. Markova IS, Berrios GE. The meaning of insight in clinical psychiatry. *Br J Psychiatry* 1992; **160**: 850–60.
7. Seltzer B, Vasterling JJ, Hale MA, Khurana R. Unawareness of memory deficit in Alzheimer's disease: relation to mood and other disease variables. *Neuropsychiatry Neuropsychol Behav Neurol* 1995; **8**(3): 176–81.
8. Eastwood R, Reisberg B. Mood and behaviour. In: Gauthier S, ed. *Clinical Diagnosis and Management of Alzheimer's Disease*. Boston, Butterworth-Heinemann. 1996; 175–89.
9. Rossor M. Alzheimer's disease. *BMJ* 1993; **307**: 779–82.
10. Cummings JL, Mega M, Gray K, *et al.* The Neuropsychiatric Inventory: comprehensive assessment of psychopathology in dementia. *Neurology* 1994; **44**: 2308–14.
11. Cummings JL, Trimble MR. *Concise Guide to Neuropsychiatry and Behavioral Neurology*. Washington, DC, American Psychiatric Press, Inc, 1995.
12. Magaziner J. Use of proxies to measure health and functional outcomes in effectiveness research in persons with Alzheimer's disease and related disorders. *Alzheimer Dis Assoc Disord* 1997; **11**(6): 168–74.
13. Zimmerman SI, Magaziner J. Methodological issues in measuring the functional status of cognitively impaired nursing home residents: the use of proxies and performance-based measures. *Alzheimer Dis Assoc Disord* 1994; **8**(1): S281–90.
14. Coen RF, O'Boyle CA, Coakley D, Lawlor BA. Dementia carer education and patient behaviour disturbance. *Int J Geriatr Psychiatry* 1999; **14**: 302–6.

15. Logsdon RG, Gibbons LE, McCurry SM, Teri L. Assessing quality of life in older adults with cognitive impairment. *Psychosom Med* 2002; **64**: 510–19.

16. Brod M, Stewart AL, Sands L, Walton P. Conceptualisation and measurement of quality of life in dementia: the Dementia Quality of Life instrument (DQoL). *Gerontologist* 1999; **39**(1): 25–35.

17. Salek MS, Schwartzberg E, Bayer AJ. Evaluating health-related quality of life in patients with dementia: development of a proxy self-administered questionnaire. *Pharm World Sci* 1996; **18**(5 Suppl A): 6.

18. Rabins P, Kasper JD, Kleinman L, Black BS, Patrick DL. Concepts and methods in the development of the ADRQL: an instrument for assessing health-related quality of life in persons with Alzheimer's disease. *J Ment Health Aging* 1999; **5**(1): 33–48.

19. DeLetter MC, Tully CL, Wilson JF, Rich EC. Nursing staff perceptions of quality of life of cognitively impaired elders: instrumental development. *J Appl Gerontol* 1995; **14**(4): 426–43.

20. World Health Organization. *WHO Meeting on the Assessment of Quality of Life in Health Care.* MNH/PSF/91.4). Geneva, WHO 1991.

21. Johnson TM. Cultural considerations. In: Spilker B, ed. *Quality of Life and Pharmacoeconomics in Clinical Trials*, 2nd edn. Philadelphia, Lippincott-Raven. 1996; 511–15.

22. Acquadro C, Jambon B, Ellis D, Marquis P. Language and translation issues. In: Spilker B, ed. *Quality of Life and Pharmacoeconomics in Clinical Trials*, 2nd edn. Philadelphia, Lippincott-Raven. 1996; 575–85.

23. Fukushima T, Nagahata K, Ishibashi N, Takahashi Y, Moriyama M. Quality of life from the viewpoint of patients with dementia in Japan: nurturing through an acceptance of dementia by patients, their families and care professionals. *Health Soc Care Community* 2005; **13**(1): 30–7.

24. Chee YK, Levkoff SE. Culture and dementia: accounts by family caregivers and health professionals for dementia-affected elders in South Korea. *J Cross Cult Gerontol* 2001; **16**(2): 111–25.

25. Hinton L, Franz CE, Yeo G, Levkoff SE. Conceptions of dementia in a multiethnic sample of family caregivers. *J Am Geriatr Soc* 2005; **53**(8): 1405–10.

26. Nightingale MC. Religion, spirituality, and ethnicity: what it means for caregivers of persons with Alzheimer's disease and related disorders. *Dementia* 2003; **2**(3): 379–91.

27. Ampil ER, Fook-Chong S, Sodagar SN, Chen CP, Auchus AP. Ethnic variability in dementia: results from Singapore. *Alzheimer Dis Assoc Disord* 2005; **19**(4): 184–5.

28. Prince M. Dementia in developing countries. A consensus statement from the 10/66 Dementia Research Group. *Int J Geriatr Psychiatry* 2000; **15**(1): 14–20.

29. Prince M, Acosta D, Chiu H, Scazufka M, Varghese M. Dementia diagnosis in developing countries: a cross-cultural validation study. *Lancet* 2003; **361**: 909–17.

30. Rajkumar S, Kumar S, Thara R. Prevalence of dementia in a rural setting: a report from India. *Int J Geriatr Psychiatry* **12**(7): 702–8.

31. World Health Organization. *The ICD-10 Classification of Mental and Behavioural Disorders. Diagnostic Criteria for Research.* Geneva, World Health Organization, 1993.

32. Rait G, Burns A. Appreciating background and culture: the South Asian elderly and mental

health. *Int J Geriatr Psychiatry* 1997; **12**(10): 973–7.

33. Regiane G, Paulo RM. Brazil is ageing: good and bad news from an epidemiological perspective. *Rev Bras Psiquiatr* 2002; **24**(1): 3–6.
34. Gilliard J, Means R, Beattie A, Daker-White G. Dementia care in England and the social model of disability: lessons and issues. *Dementia* 2005; **4**(4): 571–86.
35. Jarrott SE, Zarit SH, Berg S, Johansson L. Adult day care for dementia: a comparison of programs in Sweden and the United States. *J Cross Cult Gerontol* 1998; **13**(2): 99–108.
36. Cloutterbuck J, Mahoney DF. African American dementia caregivers: the duality of respect. *Dementia* 2003; **2**(2): 221–43.
37. Mausbach BT, Coon DW, Depp C, *et al.* Ethnicity and time to institutionalization of dementia patients: a comparison of Latina and Caucasian female family caregivers. *J Am Geriatr Soc* 2004; **52**(7): 1077–84.
38. Ganguli M, Ratcliff G, Chandra V, *et al.* A Hindi version of the MMSE: the development of a cognitive screening instrument for a largely illiterate rural elderly population in India. *Int J Geriatr Psychiatry* 1995; **10**(5): 367–77.
39. Copeland JR, Kelleher MJ, Kellett JM, *et al.* A semi-structured clinical interview for the assessment of diagnosis and mental state in the elderly: the Geriatric Mental State Schedule. I. Development and reliability. *Psychol Med* 1976; **6**(3): 439–49.

Psychosocial factors

Caregiving for dementia: global perspectives and transcultural issues

Thaddeus Alfonso, Ennapadam S. Krishnamoorthy, and Keith Gomez

Introduction

Globally the number of older persons (60 years or over) will be more than triple, increasing from 606 million today to nearly 2 billion by 2050. The increase in the number of the oldest old (80 years or over) is expected to be even more marked, passing from 69 million in 2000 to 379 million in 2050, more than a fivefold increase [1]. As the proportion of elderly is on the increase throughout the world, the number of people with dementia will increase, and this presents major healthcare problems in most societies [2,3]. Dementia is one of the most debilitating conditions to affect elderly people. It is not one person's illness alone; there is almost always a second patient in the making (the family caregiver) when a person is diagnosed with dementia [4]. In developing nations family caregivers bear the main responsibility for the people with dementia, the majority of whom continue to live at home until the very end [3]. Almost 80% of persons with dementia are cared for in their homes by family members [5]. Many studies have shown that caring for a person with dementia can have a negative effect on the caregiver's physical, psychological or emotional health, social life, and economy and is defined as caregiver burden [6–8]. The disease adversely and in some cases drastically affects the interactional patterns and role functioning of various family members in the household and also affects members of the extended family.

Caring for a relative with dementia is demanding and fraught with emotional distress, physical exhaustion, and in some cases suppressed hostility. Many previous studies have demonstrated the negative psychological, physical, and social consequences associated with providing care to a relative with Alzheimer's disease [9–11]. Caregivers are also likely to become socially isolated in some instances, because of the demanding nature

Dementia: A Global Approach, ed. Ennapadam S. Krishnamoorthy, Martin J. Prince, and Jeffrey L. Cummings. Published by Cambridge University Press.

and intensity of their caregiving role [12]. In this context, caregivers are critical focuses for intervention in their own right, as their health directly influences the patient's quality of life [12]. Thus it is imperative to provide education, training, and access to resources for the family members and other caregivers.

The caregiver

The family caregiver can be defined by the relationship (spouse, child, and professional), primacy (primary or secondary caregiver), living arrangements (with the recipient or separately), style of care (regular, occasional, and routine), and job description (formal-paid or informal-unpaid) [13]. Caregivers have been described as "hidden patients" [14]. The majority of people with dementia continue to live at home because of the unpaid assistance of family caregivers [15–18], and the stress and burden of the caregiver varies according to the stages and progression of the illness.

Impact of caring on caregivers

Family caregivers of dementia patients have an extremely high risk of developing affective disorders such as major depression and anxiety disorder [19,20]. The month prevalence of depressive disorders among caregivers varied between 15% and 32% in three representative community samples, the 12 months' incidence of depressive disorders was 48% as reported in one representative sample [20,21]. Data on anxiety disorders in dementia caregivers are scarce but suggest that one in three caregivers suffers from an anxiety disorder [22]. Depressive and anxiety symptoms are even more prevalent and affect between half and three-quarters of all caregivers [20,21,23]. The risk to develop an affective disorder persists over many years of caregiving and even after caregiving ends with the death of the care recipient [19,24].

The accumulating evidence on the personal, social, occupational, and health effects of dementia caregiving has generated a broad range of intervention studies, including randomized trials aimed at decreasing the burden and stress of caregiving. Several studies have demonstrated statistically significant effects in reducing caregiver burden, lowering caregiver depression, and delaying institutionalization of care recipients [25,26,27] through either targeted interventions that treat a specific caregiver problem, such as depression, or broad-based multicomponent interventions that include counseling, telephone support, case management, and access to resources.

Despite a wide range of useful services that can help patients and provide relief to caregivers, the burden of caregiving remains very high [17], and the caregivers' use of support services is low. Perceived lack of need and/or lack of awareness are the main reasons for this non-use of services [28]. Development and evaluation of intervention programs for family caregivers is urgently required to prevent and relieve the stress of caregiving.

Caregiver education and training: empowering the caregiver

Caregivers who receive information, advice, and support will be more able to achieve a satisfactory outcome for their relative and for themselves [9]. A number of different intervention programs have been described in the literature [26,29–31], but the content of intervention for carers of patients with dementia has varied widely. Given differing results of intervention studies, a meta-analysis of 78 studies was used to evaluate the effects on caregiver's burden, depression, subjective well-being, perceived caregiver's satisfaction, ability/knowledge and symptoms of the person in receipt of care [30]. Intervention for caregivers is more effective among elderly without dementia than caregivers of elderly with dementia. Systematic reviews and meta-analyses show that information and support alone are helpful but only address the psychological needs of caregivers modestly at best [26,30].

Programs that demonstrate beneficial effects on affective disorders involving both patients and their families are more intensive and modified to caregivers' needs [26,32]. As demonstrated in the landmark studies of Mittelman *et al.*, family meetings, designed to mobilize support of naturally existing family networks, appear to be among the most powerful psychosocial interventions to reduce depression in caregivers [33–36].

Family and caregiver counseling can maximize the positive contributions of each member to caregiving [37]; enhance the process of sharing the caregiving role; improve the caregiver's understanding of how to ask for help, what kind of help is reasonable to expect from family members, and how to accept help; and reduce family conflict. In addition, these programs resulted in postponement of nursing home placement of patients [34,38].

Psycho educational interventions include providing information on the care-receiver's disease, available resources and services, and training to respond effectively to disease-specific problems. Such interventions make use of one-to-one sessions, group sessions, lectures, and written materials and these sessions should be given to caregivers repeatedly over a number of weeks, for a couple of hours each week [39]. Sustaining the family members' multiple roles in other domains of life, particularly occupational and social, is critical to the caregiving process.

Poulshock and Deimling's [40] model of psychosocial morbidity in the caregiver is portrayed with other confounding variables in Table 7B.1.

Empirical evidence suggests that carers do well if they are rendered with some form of education or training [39,41]. Education and training is the primary goal of caregiver intervention [42] and this course could be conducted in a series of sessions with the following contents:

Table 7B.1 Exacerbating and protective factors for caregivers of dementia patients

Exacerbating factors	Dementia	Protective factors
Social isolation	Dependency and problem behaviors	Practical support
Lack of knowledge	Burden on caregivers	Family help
Maladaptive coping	**Caregiver strain**	Problem-focused coping
Poor marital relationship	Psychological, social, physical, financial	Social reserves
High expressed emotions		

Adapted from Poulshock and Deimling [40]

1. Nature, etiology, epidemiology, and prognosis of the illness;
2. Information on available treatment modalities: pharmacological and non-pharmacological;
3. Interventions for the patient and the caregiver: daily activities for patient and the caregiver; a range of psychotherapies including cognitive behavior therapy, cognitive retaining, Jacobson's progressive muscle relaxation, supportive counseling; structured family meetings; and self-help support groups [43];
4. Provision of social support systems; and
5. Information on necessary legal advice and statutory benefits, particularly financial.

The intervention would involve a range of strategies: provision of information, didactic instruction, role playing, problem solving, skills training, stress management techniques, and telephone support groups to reduce risk in the caregivers' major problem areas. Providing caregivers with education, skills to manage troublesome behaviors, social support, cognitive strategies for reframing negative emotional responses, and strategies for enhancing healthy behaviors and managing stress [44] are some of the methods employed. An empowering eclectic intervention module provided by the multidisciplinary team will ensure adequate caregiver management of the patient and reduce caregiver stress (Figure 7B.1).

Key transcultural issues

In traditional cultures like India and China it has been observed that caregivers have a low perception of distress. The predominant view of caregiving in these settings is one of "duty," "obligation" or "karma" (what can I do, it is his fate and mine is, for example, an oft-repeated

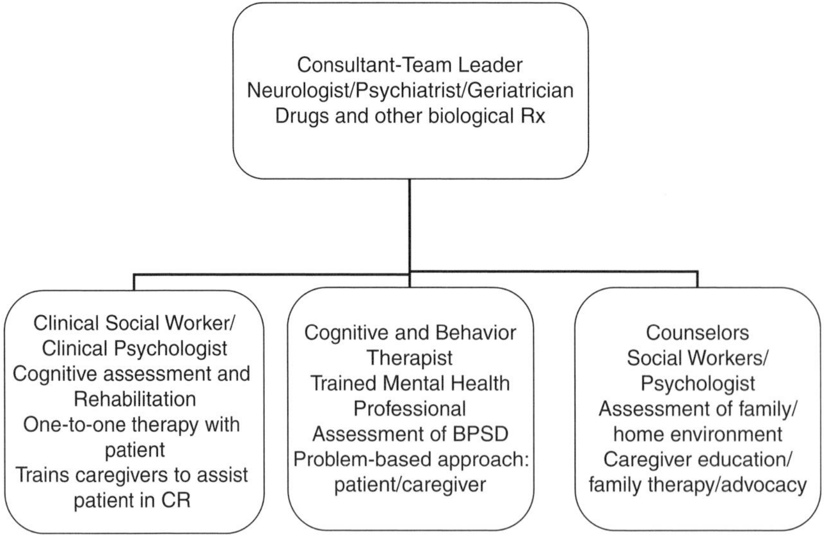

Figure 7B.1 The multidisciplinary team approach. BPSD, behavioral and psychological symptoms of dementia; CR, cognitive retraining; Rx, treatment.

phrase in India). Western commentators have alluded to this poor perception of caregiver distress being due to respect, guilt, or other social barriers preventing the caregiver from sharing true feelings. However, working with caregivers in India, we observe most commonly a failure of the caregiver to link his/her distress with the caregiving process. This agnosia for caregiver strain is in our view unlikely to be due to a conscious process. Instead it reflects a social ethos of people accustomed to adversity: one of acceptance, forbearance, and tolerance. In these societies the elder has a status that confers on her/him respect and care. Younger members of extended families and communities naturally assume many of the responsibilities of the elder (even elders who are healthy), doing their shopping, banking, and going to the post office on their behalf. Thus, the dementia caregiver in traditional societies views the caregiving that the illness necessitates as part of a natural process and while perceiving physical and emotional distress, like all caregivers elsewhere in the world, does not attribute it to the caregiving process. Clinicians and researchers working in these cultures should therefore reflect on the value of making this association for the caregiver, between the person s/he is caregiving for and her/his own symptoms. Will bringing such an association to the caregiver's consciousness truly aid the caregiving process, or will it impede it? Perhaps caregiver agnosia protects the integrity of the relationship between the person providing the care and the dementia sufferer. Perhaps professionals exposed mostly to a Western model of scientific thought and clinical training need to reflect more on the innate wisdom of these traditional cultures.

Conclusion

Dementia is a syndrome with drastic consequences for both patients and their relatives. For the carers, there is uncertainty about their family members becoming more cantankerous as they age, changing from a familiar parent or spouse into a stranger. Caregiver burden increases as the illness progresses. Previous work suggests that psychosocial issues of caregivers result from a complex interplay of factors that include characteristics of the patient and caregiver, as well as cultural factors [45–50]. Researchers suggest making the interventions available at primary, secondary, and tertiary levels. Education and training are accepted means of enhancing the carer's understanding of the illness and enriching the treatment process to improve their quality of life. This becomes a reality only when a multidisciplinary team renders those services in a well-connected and credible professional network as aging brains and minds have changing needs requiring flexible and creative responses.

References

1. World Population Prospects – The 2000 revision. United Nations Population Division. New York, NY 10017. Available at www.un.org/esa/population/unpop.htm.
2. Jacoby R, Oppenheimer C. *Psychiatry in the Elderly*. Oxford, Oxford University Press, 2002.
3. The Ministry of Health and Social Affairs. *OECD (organization for Economic Co-operation and Development) Case Study on Dementia*. Dnr S2002/7722. Stockholm, The Ministry of Health and Social Affairs (Socialdepartementet), 2004.
4. O'Brien J, Ames D, Burns A. *Dementia*. London, Arnold, 2000.

5. Haley WE. The family caregiver's role in Alzheimer's disease. *Neurology* 1997; **48**(Suppl 6): S25–9.

6. George L, Gwyther L. Caregiver well-being: a multidimensional examination of family caregivers of demented adults. *Gerontologist* 1986; **26**: 253–9.

7. Dunkin J, Anderson-Hanley C. Dementia caregiver burden: a review of the literature and guidelines for assessment and intervention. *Neurology* 1998; **51**(Suppl 1): 53–60.

8. Wimo A, Jönsson B, Karlsson I, Winblad B. *Health Economics of Dementia*. New York, John Wiley & Sons, 1998.

9. Vitaliano PP, Russo J, Young HM, Teri L, Maiuro RD. Predictors of burden in spouse caregivers of individuals with Alzheimer's disease. *Psychol Aging* 1991; **6**: 392–402.

10. Kiecolt-Glaser JK, Dura JR, Speicher CE, Trask OJ, Glaser R.. Spousal caregivers of dementia victims: longitudinal changes in immunity and health. *Psychosom Med* 1991; **53**: 345–62.

11. Brodaty H, Hadzi-Pavlovic D: Psychosocial effects on carers of living with persons with dementia. *Aust N Z J Psychiatry* 1990; **24**: 351–61.

12. Brodaty H, Luscombe G. Psychological morbidity in caregivers is associated with depression in patients with dementia. *Alzheimer Dis Assoc Disord* 1998; **12**(2): 62–70.

13. Barer BM, Johnson CL. A critique of the caregiving literature. *Gerontologist* 1990; **30**: 26–9.

14. Andolsek KM, Clapp-Channing NE, Gehlbach SH, *et al.* Caregivers and elderly relatives: the prevalence of caregiving in a family practice. *Arch Intern Med* 1988; **148**: 2177–80.

15. Arno PS, Levine C, Memmott MM. The economic value of informal caregiving. *Health Aff (Millwood).* 1999; **18**: 182–8.

16. Covinsky KE, Eng C, Lui LY, *et al.* Reduced employment in caregivers of frail elders: impact of ethnicity, patient clinical characteristics, and caregiver characteristics. *J Gerontol A Biol Sci Med Sci* 2001; **56**: M707–13.

17. Manton KG, Corder LS, Stallard E. Estimates of change in chronic disability and institutional incidence and prevalence rates in the US elderly population from the 1982, 1984, and 1989 National Long Term Care Survey. *J Gerontol* 1993; **48**: S153–66.

18. Fried LP, Guralnik JM. Disability in older adults: evidence regarding significance, etiology, and risk. *J Am Geriatr Soc* 1997; **45**: 92–100.

19. Schulz R, Beach SR. Caregiving as a risk factor for mortality: the Caregiver Health Effects Study. *JAMA* 1999; **282**: 2215–19.

20. Cuijpers P. Depressive disorders in caregivers of dementia patients: a systematic review. *Aging Ment Health* 2005; **9**: 325–30.

21. Ballard CG, Eastwood C, Gahir M, Wilcock G: A follow up study of depression in the carers of dementia sufferers. *BMJ* 1996; **312**: 947.

22. Akkerman RL, Ostwald SK. Reducing anxiety in Alzheimer's disease family caregivers: the effectiveness of a nine-week cognitive-behavioral intervention. *Am J Alzheimers Dis Other Demen* 2004; **19**: 117–123.

23. National Alliance for Caregiving and AARP *Family Caregiving in the US: Findings from a National Survey*. Washington, DC, National Alliance for Caregiving and AARP, 1997.

24. Robinson-Whelen S, Tada Y, MacCallum RC, McGuire L, Kiecolt-Glaser JK. Long-term caregiving: what happens when it ends? *J Abnorm Psychol* 2001; **110**: 573–84.

25. Schulz R, Martire LM. Family caregiving of persons with dementia: prevalence, health

effects, and support strategies. *Am J Geriatr Psychiatry* 2004; **12**: 240–9. [PMID: 15126224]

26. Brodaty H, Green A, Koschera A. Meta-analysis of psychosocial interventions for caregivers of people with dementia. *J Am Geriatr Soc* 2003; **51**: 657–64. [PMID: 12752841]
27. Schulz R, Martire LM, Klinger JN. Evidence-based caregiver interventions in geriatric psychiatry. *Psychiatr Clin North Am* 2005; **28**: 1007–38, x. [PMID: 16325738]
28. Brodaty H, Thomson C, Thompson C, Fine M. Why caregivers of people with dementia and memory loss don't use services. *Int J Geriatr Psychiatry* 2005; **20**: 537–46.
29. Collins C, Given BA, Given C. Interventions with family caregivers of persons with Alzheimer's disease. *Nurs Clin North Am* 1994; **29**: 195–207.
30. Sorensen S, Pinquart M, Duberstein P. How effective are interventions with caregivers? An updated meta-analysis. *Gerontologist* 2002; **42**: 356–72.
31. Cooke DD, McNally L, Mulligan KT, Harrison MJ, Newman SP. Psychosocial interventions for caregivers of people with dementia: a systematic review. *Aging Ment Health* 2001; **5**: 120–35.
32. Acton GJ, Winter MA. Interventions for family members caring for an elder with dementia. *Annu Rev Nurs Res* 2002; **20**: 149–79.
33. Whitlatch CJ, Zarit SH, von Eye A. Efficacy of interventions with caregivers: a reanalysis. *Gerontologist* 1991; **31**: 9–14.
34. Mittelman MS, Roth DL, Coon DW, Haley WE. Sustained benefit of supportive intervention for depressive symptoms in caregivers of patients with Alzheimer's disease. *Am J Psychiatry* 2004; **161**: 850–6.
35. Mittelman MS, Ferris SH, Shulman E, *et al.* A comprehensive support program: effect on depression in spouse-caregivers of AD patients. *Gerontologist* 1995; **35**: 792–802.
36. Mittelman MS, Ferris SH, Shulman E, Steinberg G, Levin B. A family intervention to delay nursing home placement of patients with Alzheimer disease. A randomized controlled trial. *JAMA* 1996; **276**: 1725–31.
37. Gilliard J. Counselling and alternative support for caregivers of people with dementia. Presentation at Alzheimer's Disease International Conference, Jerusalem, 1996.
38. Mittelman MS, Haley WE, Clay OJ, Roth DL. Improving caregiver well-being delays nursing home placement of patients with Alzheimer disease. *Neurology* 2006; **67**: 1592–9.
39. Brodaty H, Gresham M. Effect of a training programme to reduce stress in carers of patients with dementia. *BMJ* 1989; **299**: 1375–9.
40. Poulshock SW, Deimling GT. Families caring for elders in residence: issues in the measurement of burden. *J Gerontology* 1984; **39**: 230–9.
41. Magni E, Zanetti O, Bianchetti A, Binetti G, Trabucchi M. Evaluation of an Italian educational programme for dementia caregivers: results of a small-scale pilot study. *Int J Geriatr Psychiatry* 1995; **10**: 569–73.
42. Cummings JL, Mega MS. *Neuropsychiatry and Behavioural Neuroscience*. Oxford, Oxford University Press, 2003.
43. Toseland R, Rossiter C. Group interventions to support family caregivers: a review and analysis. *Gerontologist* 1989; **29**: 438–48.
44. REACH II. *Resources for Enhancing Alzheimer's Caregiver Health*. Pittsburgh, PA: University of Pittsburgh Epidemiology Data Center. Available at www.edc.pitt.edu/reach2/public. Last accessed on September 7, 2006.

45. Donaldson C, Tarrier N, Burns A. The impact of the symptoms of dementia on caregivers. *Br J Psychiatry* 1997; **170**: 62–8.

46. Janevic MR, Connell CM. Racial, ethnic, and cultural differences in the dementia caregiving experience: recent findings. *Gerontologist* 2001; **41**: 334–47.

47. Schulz R, O'Brien AT, Bookwala J, Fleissner K. Psychiatric and physical morbidity effects of dementia caregiving: prevalence, correlates, and causes. *Gerontologist* 1995; **35**: 771–91.

48. Schulz R, Williamson GM. A 2-year longitudinal study of depression among Alzheimer's caregivers. *Psychol Aging* 1991; **6**: 569–78.

49. Clyburn LD, Stones MJ, Hadjistavropoulos T, Tuokko H. Predicting caregiver burden and depression in Alzheimer's disease. *J Gerontol B Psychol Sci Soc Sci* 2000; **55**: S2–13.

50. Livingston G, Manela M, Katona C. Depression and other psychiatric morbidity in carers of elderly people living at home. *BMJ* 1996; **312**: 153–6.

Psychosocial factors

Care arrangements for patients with dementia: China

Helen Chiu, Joshua Tsoh, and Xin Yu

Introduction

Globally, 24 million people suffer from dementia; more than one-fifth of them reside in China [1], the world's most populous nation [2]. Formulation of care arrangements to meet their healthcare needs is a major public health challenge.

The availability of and accessibility to health care differ vastly across the 32 provinces and 2 special administrative regions of the nation; the contrast between the coastal urban areas and the less affluent rural west is especially marked. In Hong Kong, a special administrative region that returned to China's sovereignty in 1997 after a century of British colonial rule, the development of its healthcare infrastructure has followed an entirely different path from that in the mainland of China. These differences will be outlined in this chapter.

Epidemiology of dementia in Chinese populations

Representative epidemiological studies conducted in the past decade have shown that the prevalence of dementia in Chinese persons aged over 65 ranges from 2.5% to 5.9% [3–6]. Alzheimer's disease (AD) is more common than vascular dementia (VaD) or other forms of dementia; and the prevalence is similar in urban and rural areas [6]. In Hong Kong, the prevalence of dementia in those aged over 70 was 6.1%; AD accounted for 64.6% of the cases while VaD accounted for 29.3% [7]. These figures are comparable to findings in Western societies; an exponential rise in the prevalence of dementia with age is also found.

Aging in China: sociodemography

In 2006, 11% of the 1.3 billion population in China was 60 years or older. While this ratio is higher (18.2%) in large cities like Shanghai [6], the pace of population aging is faster in the rural areas of the country [8]. At 11%, the proportion of the 7 million Hong Kong citizens aged over 65 is close to the national average [9]. With a low and declining fertility rate and prolonged life expectancy, the nation is undergoing rapid

Dementia: A Global Approach, ed. Ennapadam S. Krishnamoorthy, Martin J. Prince, and Jeffrey L. Cummings. Published by Cambridge University Press.

aging. It has been forecast that by 2030, in cities like Beijing and Hong Kong, the aged population will have doubled in number [9], and nationwide, one-fifth of all inhabitants will have reached the senescence threshold.

Traditionally, the family has played a central role in the support of the elderly; less than 10% of the elderly in China live alone [10]. In Beijing and Shanghai, individuals with dementia are looked after mainly by their relatives at home (96.3% and 87.3% respectively) [11,12]. However, nationwide the size of the average household is fast dwindling (the 1% National Population Sample Survey in 2005 reported that the average family size was 3.1; down from 3.7 in 1995) [13]. This is probably due to a myriad of factors including the one-child policy, the tendency for the younger generation to migrate from rural areas into the cities, or to move from governmental dormitories to new apartments, leaving the aged parents behind, and the social and economic forces in the last decades that have led to the erosion of "filial piety" [6,14]. Indeed in Hong Kong, even more (25%) of the elderly live without their children [15].

Care arrangements for dementia: mainland China

Medical services are a constituent part of the social welfare system in China [6]. Around 5.5% of the gross domestic product (GDP) per capita (around US$800 in 2000) is devoted to healthcare expenses, but 80% of the resources are concentrated in big cities that are inhabited by 15% of the population [8]. There have been recent reforms in China to move from a fully state-financed health system to a state-subsidized health system, but the current generation of elderly lived their adulthood in a "planned economy" and have very limited savings for their healthcare expenses after retirement. The government pension system barely covers one-fifth of the country's retirees. Private medical insurance, gaining popularity nationwide, is unaffordable for most retirees [8]. It is noteworthy that most of the private health insurance companies do not provide insurance for people over 60. This policy would be regarded as ageist and discriminatory in many developed countries, but is generally accepted in China.

Specialist care for dementia

Psychogeriatric services in China are expanding but there is an ever-growing demand. At present, the availability of inpatient services and trained personnel is still limited. In 1997 only 10% of the beds in the nation's 485 psychiatric hospitals serviced the elderly [6]. In a survey published in 2006, the rate had increased to 61% [16] but this translated into only 0.06–2.2 beds per 10 000 elderly persons. The beds were mostly concentrated in big cities like Shanghai (2.2 per 10 000) and Beijing (0.97 per 10 000). Around 40% of these inpatients suffered from dementia [16].

Besides geriatric psychiatrists, other doctors also look after patients with dementia. In fact, in China most patients with dementia will visit neurologists or traditional Chinese medical physicians, if they seek treatment. It is estimated that up to 70% of patients with dementia are under the care of neurologists. In general, patients with severe dementia or those with behavioral and psychological dysfunction are more likely to see psychiatrists.

In 2006, there were only 0.03 qualified psychogeriatricians per 10 000 elderly persons. The rate was highest in Shanghai (0.15 per 10 000) and Beijing (0.12 per 10 000); in Guangdong, the rate was only 1 in 1 million [16,17].

Primary care for dementia

Physicians in primary care generally have limited training in dementia and related care; it was reported that only one-fourth of patients with dementia were correctly identified by the attending physician, and significantly fewer were referred for related therapies [16,17]. Moreover, a referral system to seek secondary and tertiary medical care is not yet in place [6].

In the rural areas where most of the elderly live, traditional Chinese medical practitioners provide approximately one-third of outpatient and one-quarter of inpatient care [8]. A pension or old age allowance is nearly non-existent [8]. Physicians are often less intensively trained [8], and there has been no systematic reporting of the care arrangements for rural dwellers with dementia in the literature.

However, the improvement of medical resources in rural areas has become the state's priority, as outlined in the "Ninth Five Year Plan for National Economic and Social Development and Long-Range Objectives to the Year 2010." It is proposed that the three-tiered medical service network in county, township, and village be consolidated. The state-subsidized cooperative medical services (CMS) providing basic medical services to rural dwellers will be strengthened [18].

Residential care

Nursing homes for the aged are in increasing demand with the stated rising dementia population and diminishing intergenerational support. However, the current number of available bed spaces (1.04 million) corresponds to less than 1% of the total elderly population in China. Nursing homes are often located in remote areas and unaffordable for most families, and many of them are of substandard quality in staffing and equipment, especially for dementia care [6,10]. In fact, almost all nursing homes refuse to admit the elderly with dementia since nursing homes which are run for profit are reluctant to make the necessary effort and arrangements for dementia care, while welfare nursing homes cannot afford to do it. More recently, non-governmental organizations (NGOs) such as the Chinese Federation for the Disabled and Handicapped have increased their contribution to build nursing homes for poorly functioning elderly people (including the elderly with dementia) [6].

Community services

For the majority of relatives who need to take care of the elderly with dementia at home, the current provision of community support is generally limited [6]. A "family bed" system exists in certain regions, providing medical treatment and nursing care for patients living at home. It caters for patients who have difficulty receiving hospitalization or need a long period of post-discharge care. The system also caters for the elderly with dementia, and relieves somewhat the burden of hospitalization [19]. "Nursemaids" are hired by families to take care of bedridden old people at home or at hospital [10].

In Beijing and other major cities, there are additional community services for debilitated elderly, which include volunteers, hot-line services, and meals-on-wheels [19].

Care arrangements for dementia: Hong Kong

In Hong Kong, 5.7% of the GDP per capita of US$26 400 is spent on health care. While 85% of primary care is provided by private practitioners, tertiary care is provided primarily by the government at a nominal fee to the user.

Adapted from the Nottingham model in the UK, specialized psychogeriatric services commenced in 1991, and rapid development in the field has taken place in the last few years [20]. Currently most of the specialist care for dementia is provided by psychogeriatricians, while geriatricians more commonly treat elderly with VaD, especially those with comorbid physical problems. At present, there are seven multidisciplinary psychogeriatric teams delivering inpatient, outpatient, day patient, outreach, and consultation-liaison services to patients in their respective geographical cluster (each with around 100 000 citizens aged over 65). In 2006, the number of fully trained psychogeriatricians and the number of day hospital places and inpatient beds designated for elderly with mental conditions stood at 0.27, 1.7, and 4.2 per 10 000 elderly persons respectively.

Community and residential care

The community psychogeriatric team serviced by psychiatrists and nurses attends to the homes for the aged and nursing homes within the catchment areas of the teams to provide domiciliary assessment and treatment of psychogeriatric patients. Close working relationships are maintained with various agencies involved in elderly care, particularly the Social Welfare Department of the Hong Kong Government and NGOs.

Community support services are mainly provided by NGOs and subsidized by the government. They provide daycare centers, home help and home rehabilitative services, and residential care. The elderly in Hong Kong are also entitled to old age allowance, and there is a range of subsidies for disabilities, diseases, unemployment, and long-term residential care.

Residential services include hostels for the elderly, homes for the aged, care and attention homes, and nursing homes in order of increasing degree of care/dependency. Private homes account for over half of all residential care places. The rate of institutionalization of the elderly with dementia in Hong Kong is relatively high compared with other Chinese cities [7]. Due to the heterogeneity in quality standards and training of personnel in dementia care, residential services are the emerging focus of dementia care in Hong Kong.

Legal aspects

Legal guardians can be appointed for dementia patients under the law of mainland China (not applicable in Hong Kong) to deal with their civil matters (e.g., handling of assets, testamentary capacity). In Hong Kong, a Guardianship Board to appoint guardians to make decisions on behalf of mentally incapacitated persons was set up in accordance with the Mental Health (Amendment) Ordinance in 1997. Enduring power of attorney is available but it does not cover healthcare issues. A consultation paper on the premise of advance directives has just been released.

Public education and advocacy

The *Alzheimer's Disease of China* regularly organizes public education campaigns, including commemorations for World Alzheimer's Disease Day [6].

In Hong Kong, the Alzheimer's Disease Association was set up in 1995, and the Hong Kong Psychogeriatric Association was established in 1998. Among their objectives are the facilitation of training, public awareness, and advocacy for dementia.

Care arrangements for dementia: the future

In both mainland China [8] and Hong Kong there is likely to be a gradual shift from a government-funded to a health insurance-based system to ensure financial sustainability, in the face of the soaring demand for health services. A comprehensive governmental policy on services for an aging population with increasing need for dementia care is vital. Community services for the elderly and their caregivers should be expanded to enable people with dementia to stay at home with their families. Apart from its moral underpinnings, "aging-in-place" should also represent an affordable and practical solution to the long-term care of people with dementia. The disparity in distribution of resources between rural and urban areas is a priority to be addressed. Training of primary care doctors, specialists and other healthcare professionals, as well as the development of end-of-life care are indispensable components of solutions to this enormous public health challenge.

References

1. Ferri CP, Prince M, Brayne C, *et al.* Global prevalence of dementia: a Delphi consensus study. *Lancet* 2005; **366**(9503): 2112–17.
2. World Health Organization *The World Health Report 2006 – Working Together for Health.* Geneva, World Health Organization, 2006.
3. Zhang ZX, Zahner GE, Roman GC, *et al.* Dementia subtypes in China: prevalence in Beijing, Xian, Shanghai, and Chengdu. *Arch Neurol* 2005; **62**(3): 447–53.
4. Zhou B, Hong Z, Huang M. [Prevalence of dementia in Shanghai's urban and rural areas.] *Zhonghua Liu Xing Bing Xue Za Zhi* 2001; **22**(5): 368–71.
5. Zhou DF, Wu CS, Qi H, *et al.* Prevalence of dementia in rural China: impact of age, gender and education. *Acta Neurol Scand* 2006; **114**(4): 273–80.
6. Yu X. Services to people with dementia: a worldwide view – China. In: Burns A, O'Brien J, Ames D, eds. *Dementia.* London, Hodder Arnold. 2005; 261–4.
7. Chiu HF, Lam LC, Chi I, *et al.* Prevalence of dementia in Chinese elderly in Hong Kong. *Neurology* 1998; **50**(4): 1002–9.
8. Woo J, Kwok T, Sze FK, Yuan HJ. Ageing in China: health and social consequences and responses. *Int J Epidemiol* 2002; **31**(4): 772–5.
9. Census and Statistics Department. *Population and Vital Events.* Hong Kong, Government of the Hong Kong Special Administrative Region, 2006.
10. Ineichen B. Influences on the care of demented elderly people in the People's Republic of China. *Int J Geriatr Psychiatry* 1998; **13**(2): 122–6.

11. He YL, Zhang MY, Qiu JY. The mental health status of dementia caregivers. *Chin J Clin Psychol* 1995; **3**: 200–4.
12. Li Y, Chen C, Luo H. The psychological well-being of caregivers of elderly dementia. *Chin Ment Health J* 1990; **4**(1): 5.
13. Chinese National Bureau of Statistics. *Statistical Report on 2005 1% National Population Sample Survey of China*. Beijing, CNSB, 2006.
14. Pochagina O. The aging of the population in the PRC: sociocultural and sociopsychological aspects. *Far East Stud* 2003; **31**(2): 79–95.
15. Phillips DR, Eh AGO. *Environment and Ageing: Environmental Policy, Planning and Design for Elderly People in Hong Kong*. Hong Kong, Centre of Urban Planning and Environmental Management, University of Hong Kong, 1999.
16. Xue HB, Yu X, Xiao SF, Zhang MY. Evaluation of the present status of psychiatric services in elderly in China. *J Clin Psychol Med* 2006; **16**(1): 11–13.
17. Ministry of Health. *The Chinese Guidelines for Dementia Therapies*. Beijing, Government of the People's Republic of China, 2006.
18. Chen MZ. *Yearbook of Health in the People's Republic of China 1997*. Beijing, The People's Medical Publishing House, 1997.
19. Chiu H, Zhang M. Services for dementia in the developing world: A Chinese view. In: O'Brien J, Ames D, Burns A, eds. *Dementia*. London, Arnold. 2000; 344–8.
20. Chiu HF, Ng LL, Nivataphand R, *et al.* Psychogeriatrics in South-East Asia. *Int J Geriatr Psychiatry* 1997; **12**(10): 989–94.

Service delivery and management

Dementia services: developing rural and remote services

Sadanand Rajkumar and Julia Lane

Dementia remains one of the most disabling and burdensome group of health conditions worldwide. Significant number of the people with dementia live in the developing world with China, India, and Latin America having the biggest increase. A major part of the populations in these regions are rural.

Countries such as China and India have 70% of the populations in rural areas where there is a demographic transition taking place, with young people both dwindling in numbers and not being available for caring for the elderly and migrating for their future job opportunities to urban settings (see Chapter 7C on caregiving). This epidemiological and demographic change will have a profound effect on caregiving and developing rural services for those with dementia.

A pre-requisite of care for dementia is the accurate diagnosis, the type and stage of dementia; the accompanying symptoms; the challenging problems of behavioral and psychological symptoms of dementia (BPSD). Complex physical, psychological, and social circumstances surround people with dementia. This chapter covers the broad issues relating to developing dementia services in rural and remote settings. A starting point in dementia care can be developed on the lines of guidelines demonstrated by the World Health Organization for mental health care in elderly, referred to by the acronym "CARITAS" [1], which aims for *comprehensive*, *accessible*, *responsive*, *individualized*, *transdisciplinary*, *accountable*, and *systemic* service delivery. Clearly, rural and remote service delivery poses certain challenges in meeting particular domains of these best practice ideals.

Accessible services present a challenge in rural and remote areas. A major obstacle to accessing timely and appropriate care is geographical distance and terrain, but other barriers include financial, cultural, and linguistic problems. Geographical distance from health and service providers may be compounded by poor-quality roads, lack of public

Dementia: A Global Approach, ed. Ennapadam S. Krishnamoorthy, Martin J. Prince, and Jeffrey L. Cummings. Published by Cambridge University Press.

transportation, or access to private vehicle, and the possible need for overnight accommodation, resulting in a financial burden. Even in circumstances where transportation exists, the patient is likely to require the escort of a carer to negotiate travel and attendance at appointments. Language barriers also exist. Professional healthcare interpreters are scarce, hence this role defaults to carers or available staff members who speak the patient's language but have no formal training. Interpreters also have an important role as "culture brokers," assisting the care provider to understand the patient's experience through the lens of their unique cultural beliefs and experiences. Research has shown that while acute crisis service usage in rural areas mirrors that in urban regions, the use of chronic care and prevention services is clearly lower. This suggests rural residents are not making the best use of existing services for the ongoing care and monitoring needed during the course of dementia, let alone being affected by the current public health emphasis on health promotion, illness prevention, early detection, and intervention [2].

Most urban areas have a comprehensive range of services available for those with dementia and their carers – this is far from the case in rural and remote regions. Ideally the spectrum of professional services available in dementia care includes the primary care physician, allied health professionals such as psychologists and social workers; occupational, diversional, and speech therapists; and nursing staff. Given the coexisting health conditions, dieticians, dentists, consultant physicians, psychiatrists and neurologists, and a range of volunteers are needed in planning services, all of whom cannot be rurally based but made available in large regional centers or districts. Rural and remote areas have a history of difficulty in attracting and retaining appropriately trained, skilled, and experienced staff. Professional isolation, heavy workloads, lack of leave cover, and "burnout" are the main difficulties. Thus, the number and range of health professionals is reduced, and they provide a service for a vast geographical area.

The range of support services and care settings available for dementia care in rural and remote areas is problematic. Although the need exists for day care, day hospitals, domiciliary support, respite, residential aged care facilities, inpatient beds, and outpatient clinics, the reduced population density and geographical spread necessitate economies of scale, i.e., not every village will have all these services on site. Whereas in an urban setting these supports enable the person with dementia to remain at home, an isolated elder living in a remote area may be institutionalized prematurely due to the lack of such services in their community. This infringes on the *Individualized* principle, which states the need for care to be tailored to each individual and their family, to meet their needs and keep people at home as long as possible. In developing countries few such community services exist, resulting in a family member assuming the role of full-time carer instead of being a paid member of the workforce. As the population ages this has a significant economic and workforce implication.

In rural areas, staff members from various agencies develop close links with each other, which facilitate communication and cooperation and help in enhancing care. On the positive side, there is little scope for duplication or fragmentation of services [3].

The *Transdisciplinary* principle highlights the need for services to transcend traditional boundaries between disciplines to maximize input from all team members. The exigencies of practicing in rural and remote areas require that staff and service providers go beyond narrow professional boundaries in order to meet the patient's needs, given the lack of availability and access to a multidisciplinary team. Primary care practitioners and community nurses have a pivotal role in the provision of health care, support for carers, and in referral to other service providers as needed.

People living in rural and remote areas are often known in their local communities, and to service providers, from before their illness onset. This knowledge and respect of the patient as a person, with a unique history, personality and social network, reflect the community cohesion present in rural communities and is a significant strength. It demonstrates the principle of comprehensive service, i.e., patient-centered and holistic in approach, taking into account the patient's biopsychosocial needs and preferences.

The *Responsive and Accountable* service seeks to understand the patients' and carers' needs and acts to meet these in a timely and appropriate manner, ensuring high-quality service provision through ongoing monitoring. A challenge for rural and remote service providers of dementia care is the provision of a broad range of best practice services despite the reduced availability of trained, skilled staff, access problems especially geographical obstacles, limited funding, and fatalistic community attitudes that perceive cognitive and functional problems as an expected and understandable part of aging.

Solutions to these problems include innovative and flexible approaches to service delivery, such as:

1. Multimedia education of the general community, patients and carers, and staff regarding dementia.
2. Practical workshops addressing day-to-day issues such as personal care and BPSD.
3. Recruitment of volunteers to assist carers and provide respite.
4. Clearer pathways to care and referral/assessment protocols.
5. Partnership agreements between services.
6. Use of technology such as telemedicine for clinical assessment, case conferencing, education, and supervision.
7. Twenty-four-hour telephone lines for advice and support.
8. Outreach clinics.

The *Systemic* principle holds that available services should be coordinated and integrated at multiple levels to provide continuity of care for the person with dementia. The rural and remote dementia services that do exist tend to be open and inclusive in their approach, attempting to work productively and cooperatively to provide a network dementia care, and consulting and referring as required. Underlying this principle in rural and remote areas is the need for more funding and advocacy for better support for the patients, families, and carers. This needs to be firmly placed on the health and political agendas. This suggests rural residents are not making the best use of existing services for dementia, given the level of ongoing care and monitoring needed during the disease course. The impact of current public emphasis, health promotion, illness prevention, early detection, and intervention is likely to be therefore lower in these populations. One model of care will not fit all, and urban models do not always translate to a rural or remote context.

Rational steps in delivery and organization of care for dementia ought to have a comprehensive approach involving the community, carers, the non-governmental organizations, and where possible the consumer. Planning of dementia care in rural settings should keep in view the strengths and limitations of rural life and be culturally sensitive, cost-effective, and replicable. Care needs to enhance the dignity and equality of those with dementia and the caregiver.

References

1. World Health Organization. *Organization of Care in Psychiatry of the Elderly – A Technical Consensus Statement.* WHO/MSA/MNH/MND/97.3. Geneva, WHO, 1997.
2. Tomlinson E, McDonagh MK, Crooks KB, Lees M. Health beliefs of rural Canadians: implications for practice. *Aust J Rural Health* 2004; **12**: 258–63.
3. Neese JN. Rural service delivery. In: Draper B, Melding P, Brodaty H, eds. *Psychogeriatric Service Delivery.* Oxford, Oxford University Press. 2005; 281–92.

Service delivery and management

Non-pharmacological approaches: patient-centered approaches

S. Kalyanasundaram

Introduction

The management of dementia should ideally combine medication and non-pharmacological management. The latter should include giving appropriate information to caregivers, addressing needs of family members, and providing emotional and psychological support. Proper guidance needs to be provided to family members at different stages of the disease and should form part of the management strategy. Issues that need to be addressed as part of this management strategy include those involving the activities of daily living, behavioral management, and attempts to improve cognitive deficits.

Utilizing primary carers

Cummings in his study [1] found family members to be "necessary partners in the planning process and as invaluable resources to discharged dementia patients." Simms *et al.* [2] suggest that patients, families, and carers should be consulted at "all points of seamless care from entry into point of service to discharge." Bull and coworkers' [3] qualitative research study, concerning the perceptions of caregivers of their involvement in the discharge process, found that the role of family and caregivers in the acute setting is fundamental in guiding nurse practice. This is based upon the finding that in those families most involved in the discharge planning process, the level of functional ability, independence, and satisfaction was higher than in those families who reported little involvement in the planning phase of discharge.

Educating the family

Educating the family about the disease, the prognosis, available treatment, and the limitations of medical management should form part of the treatment plan. Many family members find it difficult to accept and acknowledge the fact that their loved one may be suffering from dementia. Many a time, denial results in not

Dementia: A Global Approach, ed. Ennapadam S. Krishnamoorthy, Martin J. Prince, and Jeffrey L. Cummings. Published by Cambridge University Press.

seeking help at the early stages of the disease. The physician needs to take time to explain in detail the nature of the illness and this may take two to three sessions. Some family members blame themselves for not recognizing it early enough and wonder whether their own lack of interest, ignorance, and indifference may have resulted in this disease.

Counseling the family

Dementia is an illness that affects the entire family. Family counseling therefore should form an essential part of the treatment plan. It is disheartening for a family member to see someone close to them deteriorate in front of their eyes and become a shadow of their former self. If the burden is not shared by all the members of a family, the distress of the caregiver is a lot more. Counseling regarding the need to share such distress should form part of the therapeutic intervention. Psychotherapy, stress reduction programs, and the taking of short breaks to recharge themselves are certain methods that may be suggested to the caregivers.

Non-pharmacological patient-centered approaches

Despite several advances in pharmacological management in the recent years, the cure of dementia remains elusive. Further, pharmacological management alone cannot resolve the gamut of issues that affect patients with dementia and their families, and the need to combine non-pharmacological approaches remains. These non-pharmacological management strategies should be tailor-made for each individual. Although some of what will be described may not be applicable to all people with dementia, the methods employed would need to take into account the stage of the disease, associated behavioral and psychological symptoms, and the level of caregiver support that is available. It also must be understood that, despite best efforts, the outcome may not be very satisfactory to the caregivers, given the nature of the illness and the non-cooperation which one may encounter from the patients. However, these strategies must be pursued in all the patients, as even a small improvement may make a considerable difference to patient and caregiver quality of life (see also Chapter 7A on quality of life) and in most instances may offer some relief to the families.

Exercise

Regular exercise, however minimal it may be, has a place in the management of people with dementia. Many can be trained to perform simple repetitive exercises, which allow for better blood circulation, and helps to prevent falls and fractures [4,5].

Therapeutic activities and creative arts therapies

Therapeutic activities and the creative arts therapies have been recognized as beneficial, especially in persons with dementia living in long-term care facilities. Therapeutic programming emphasizes a balance of group and individual activities that promote strengths, personal interests, and abilities, as well as accomplishments, and the opportunity for self-expression. Creative arts therapies include music, art, dance/movement, drama, and bibliotherapy (literature and poetry) [6,7].

Therapeutic touch

An ancient intervention that has recently gained popularity in the field of health care is the use of therapeutic touch. In a survey of nursing home management of disruptive behavior, a little more than one-third of the staff listed touch as an intervention that provided benefit to some clients [8].

Scheduling activities of daily life

As one would expect, activities of daily living get severely compromised in patients with dementia. Caregivers automatically assume the tasks once handled by the patients. Basic daily activities such as brushing, bathing, dressing, and grooming all tend to get affected at different stages of the disease. Toileting also gets affected as the disease advances. One can approach this problem in two ways.

1. The patient could be reminded by someone else to do these tasks. If this is not sufficient, reminders should be followed by supervision. Positive reinforcement for the tasks accomplished by the patient, however small, is likely to reinforce good behavior and enhance chances of its continuing.
2. A chart with simple labels or symbols could be placed in a prominent position for the patient to see; the patient should be encouraged to view the chart frequently. Daily activities like taking a bath, medicines, and food, etc. can be thus scheduled, if reminding alone is inadequate for the patient to initiate an activity.

Physical restraint

Physical restraint does produce adverse and harmful effects especially in the elderly. Immobility causes decreased muscle mass, which results in weakness, loss of balance and, along with bone demineralization, increases the risk of falls and fractures. Additionally, the metabolic rate slows, and circulatory responses can include decreased cardiac output, increased risk of blood clots, and orthostatic hypotension.

Reality orientation

Reality orientation (RO) was developed in the United States in the 1960s. It is a basic technique used to rehabilitate persons having some form of memory loss, confusion, and disorientation in time, place, and person. Reality orientation, however, is beneficial only as long as the patient has the capacity to retain current information [9].

Validation therapy

Validation therapy was developed by Naomi Feil in 1982. It is an individual and group intervention program that focuses on the emotional content of what someone is saying rather than the factual content. The therapist validates what someone is saying by acknowledging the emotion(s) being expressed by the person. This type of therapy has been observed to work especially well with memory-impaired persons such as those with dementia [10]. Validation techniques have also been supported by Drijfhout [11] and Johns and Gurnett [12] who suggest that there is logic behind all behavior, including the disorientated behavior of patients with dementia.

Johns and Gurnett [12] in their paper describe stages of disorientation and appropriate validation therapy methods at each stage. They report that validation techniques often restore meaning and self-respect to a patient with dementia, whilst relieving emotional turmoil that is often found in the acute setting.

Pet therapy in dementia

Although the introduction of pets into nursing homes is believed to help the mood state of residents, there are very few controlled data on this issue. A preliminary study suggested utility for pet therapy in decreasing irritable behavior [13]. In addition to the paucity of controlled data, it remains unclear how patients who do not appreciate pets react to their introduction into the facility.

Music therapy

Exposure to music has been used to deal with agitation in dementia patients with variable degrees of success. Individualized music therapy intervention using music that the patient had liked and enjoyed prior to the development of illness has been found to decrease behavioral disturbances. The efficacy of music therapy has been investigated with individuals suffering from Alzheimer's disease and Aldridge [14] and Brotons and Pickett-Cooper [15] found that it is an effective treatment.

Reminiscence and life review

The concept of reviewing one's life has been shown to be a positive form of placing one's past experiences in proper perspective. It is believed to work through unresolved conflicts [16]. Empirical trials have been conducted using reminiscence and life review to reduce depression and anxiety and to increase feelings of self-esteem and life satisfaction in the elderly.

Individual case management

Most methods of case management are based on operant conditioning, contingency management, and token economy and retraining. Other approaches are counseling the carers, respite care in the form of day care, sitting care, relief care, etc. Environmental intervention involves modifying the environment, stimulus control, use of exaggerated cues, and behavioral prosthetics. Support groups, self-help groups, and Alzheimer's societies also provide help to carers.

Conclusion

A range of non-pharmacological therapies have therefore been described in the care of dementia. While randomized controlled trial level evidence is seldom available, empirical evidence suggests their utility in the care of the dementia sufferer. A holistic approach, with the appropriate use of medication, combined with individualized non-pharmacological therapy may be best placed to offer relief to the patient and thus support the caregiver.

References

1. Cummings S. Adequacy of discharge plans and rehospitalization among hospitalized dementia patients. *Health Soc Work* 1999; **24**(4): 249.

2. Simms L, Coeling H, Rosemann M. An action approach to redesigning a patient-centred unit. *Int Nurs Rev* 1998; **45**(2): 58–60.

3. Bull M, Hansen H, Gross C. Differences in family caregiver outcomes by their level of involvement in discharge planning. *Appl Nurs Res* 2000; **13**(2): 76–82.

4. Buchner DM, Larson EB. Falls and fractures in patients with Alzheimer-type dementia. *JAMA* 1987; **257**: 1492–5.

5. Myers AH, Robbinson EG, van Natta ML, *et al.* Hip fractures among the elderly: factors associated with inhospital mortality. *Am J Epidemiol* 1991; **134**: 1128–37.

6. Dalley T. (ed.) *Art as Therapy: An Introduction to the Use of Art as a Therapeutic Technique.* London, Tavistock/ Routledge, 1984.

7. Payne H. (ed.) *Dance Movement Therapy: Theory and Practice.* London, Routledge, 1992.

8. Whall AL, Gillis GL, Yankou D, *et al.* Disruptive behavior in elderly nursing home staff. *J Gerontol Nurs* 1992; **18**: 13–17.

9. Mintzer JE, Mirski DF, Hoernig KS. Behavioral and psychological signs and symptoms of dementia: a practicing psychiatrist's view point. *Dialogues Clin Neurosci* 2000; **2**(2): 139–55.

10. Devanand DP, Lawlor BA. *Treatment of Behavioural and Psychological Symptoms in Dementia.* London, Martin Dunitz, 2000.

11. Drijfhout J. Caring for people with dementia. *N Z Nursing J* 1998; **4**(8): 12–13.

12. Johns A, Gurnett A. Validating the needs of the confused elderly. *N Z Nursing J* 1998; **4**(8): 18–21.

13. Zisselman MH, Rovner BW, Shmuely Y, Ferrie P. A pet therapy intervention with geriatric psychiatry inpatients. *Am J Occup Ther* 1996; **50**: 47–51.

14. Aldridge D. Music therapy and the treatment of Alzheimer's disease. *J Clin Geropsychol* 1998; **4**(1): 17–30.

15. Brotons M, Pickett-Cooper P. The effects of music therapy intervention on agitation behaviors of Alzheimer's disease patients. *J Music Ther* 1996; **33**(1): 2–18.

16. Butler RN. The life review: an interpretation of reminiscence in the aged. *Psychiatry* 1963; **26**: 65–76.

Chapter 9A

The clinical approach to the person with dementia

Peru (South America)

Mariella Guerra

Peru is a developing country in South America in a period of demographic transition. Peru has 28 million inhabitants, 49.8% of whom live in conditions of poverty. Life expectancy at birth is 71.2 years and elderly people (aged 60 years and over) constitute 7.7% of the population. The trend is for this percentage to increase and consequently for a greater prevalence of chronic age-related disorders such as dementia [1].

Prior to the 10/66 Dementia Research Group study, there had been no other population-based studies of dementia in Peru. However, two important epidemiological mental health studies had been carried out in Peru by the National Institute of Mental Health "Honorio Delgado - Hideyo Noguchi" [2]. In both, part of the survey was focused on the mental health of older people, those aged 60 years and over. One of the topics they examined was that of cognitive functioning among elderly individuals, surveys being carried out both in coastal cities and in the highlands in years 2002 and 2003 respectively. One thousand one hundred and seventy-two elderly people were evaluated using the Mini-Mental State Examination (MMSE) as a measure of cognitive function. More people in the highlands (50%) had cognitive impairment as measured by the MMSE when compared to the coastal cities (21.5%). This high prevalence of cognitive impairment in the highlands led them to divide the sample in two: those with eight years of education and over and those with less than eight years and to reanalyze the results. Remarkably this led to a sea change in the results; only 10% of those with eight years or more of education had cognitive impairment in the coast and 8% in the highlands, with the same criteria being applied. On the other hand, cognitive impairment was higher in those with less than eight years of education; 33% in the coast and 65% in the highlands. Premorbid education in Peru (as in other parts of the world, see China [Chapter 9F] for example) is generally found to be strongly associated (positively) with cognitive function measured later in life [3]. Further, cognitive impairment is strongly associated with lower

Dementia: A Global Approach, ed. Ennapadam S. Krishnamoorthy, Martin J. Prince, and Jeffrey L. Cummings. Published by Cambridge University Press.

educational attainment or lower duration of formal education.

The implications for clinical practice in Peru are the need to keep premorbid education firmly in mind in diagnosing dementia. The diagnosis of dementia has to be made with the greatest caution in those with fewer than eight years of formal education. Caution is also required in the ready use of Western screening and diagnostic measures which have a strong educational bias.

As part of an international research effort following the 10/66 Dementia Research Group's study protocol and algorithms, a population-based survey was carried out in Peru between 2006 and 2007. A group of instruments already validated in 10/66 pilot studies for dementia diagnosis were applied by trained interviewers to 2000 elderly (aged 65 years and over)[4]. One thousand four hundred and thirty-one were from urban area and 569 from rural area. As per the 10/66 dementia diagnosis algorithm, the prevalence of dementia in the urban sample was 9.4% compared with just 6.5% in the rural sample. The prevalence of dementia was generally lower in males than in females. The prevalence of 10/66 dementia (as in other 10/66 samples around the globe) was higher than that for DSM-IV diagnosis criteria. The severity profile of dementia cases differ by area; mild cases constituting 45% of the urban sample and 30% of the rurals sample. On the other hand, severe cases of dementia formed 10% of urban sample and 6% of the rural sample surveyed.

These findings mirror clinical practice experience in Peru. As in many developing nations there is a considerable difference between urban and rural populations. The lifestyle, cultural factors, and social networks that persist in rural areas are often less prominent in urban regions (see Chapter 7B on care arrangements) with milder forms of dementia being more easily diagnosed in the urban areas. Other factors that may aid dementia diagnosis in urban as opposed to rural areas include greater awareness of cognitive impairment not being part of normal aging and greater perceived disability due to living arrangements that prevail in the urban regions.

With respect to risk factors, the Peruvian sample was characterized by low blood pressure levels and low prevalence of smoking and stroke. The variables positively associated with dementia were: female gender; small skull circumference; as reported in other studies, family history of dementia; head injury with loss of consciousness; and meat consumption.

Other aspects evaluated were factors relating to the care of the patient with dementia. This survey showed that in Peru living alone or living only with the spouse are very uncommon arrangements for people with dementia (see Table 9A.1). Children are most frequently identified as the main caregivers (see Table 9A.2) (see also Chapters 9B and 7C on approach to dementia in Nigeria and caregiving in China, respectively). Paid carers are

Table 9A.1 Living arrangements of people with dementia in Peru

	Urban %	Rural %
Alone	1.6	13.9
Spouse only	4.3	8.3
With children	29.4	41.6
Other	51.2	30.6

Table 9A.2 Who provides care for people with dementia in Peru

	Urban %	Rural %
Spouse	13	16.7
Child	40.3	55.6
Daughter- or Son-in-law	1.3	2.8
Non-relative	30	2.8
Female carer	83.7	86.1

Table 9A.3 Care arrangements for people with dementia in Peru

	Urban %	Rural %
Cut back on work to care	6.2	11.1
Additional informal unpaid care	27.1	19.4
Paid care day	22.5	2.8
Paid care night	15.6	2.8

commonly employed in Peru and cutting back on work to care is not usual in urban areas (see Table 9A.3) (see Chapter 1). Caregiver strain also was evaluated. Levels were as high as those typically seen in developed country studies. Zarit burden interview (adjusted for diferent variables) was 15.5 for the urban area and 18.6 for the rural one. Dementia by itself is a risk factor for depression in the carer and is worst if it is associated with behavioral and psychological dysfunction in line with reports from elsewhere.

Table 9A.4 Pension and welfare arrangements for people with dementia in Peru

	Government or occupational pension %	Disability pension %	Family transfer %
Urban	58.9	0.8	4.7
Rural	66.7	0.0	0.0

Table 9A.5 Health service use (last three months) by people with dementia in Peru

	Primary care %	Private doctor %	No services %
Urban	5.5	8.6	58.9
Rural	19.4	11.1	41.7

Table 9A.4 gives a welfare approach. It seems to be that a great number of dementia patients are covered with a pension but disability pensions are generally not available for people with dementia (0.8% urban, 0.0% rural).

Finally an important issue is that related to health service use. In contrast to physical conditions, dementia is not associated with receiving health services. Most people with dementia in Peru have used no healthcare services in the last three months (see Table 9A.5).

The implications of these findings are that dementia is an important and emerging public health problem in Peru with important rural/urban differences in prevalence, severity, caregiving, and service utilization.

References

1. Instituto Nacional de Estadística e Informática. Perú: Estimaciones y Proyecciones de Población, 1950–2050. Lima, INEA, 2001.

2. Instituto Nacional de Salud Mental "Honorio Delgado - Hideyo Noguchi". Estudio Epidemiológico Metropolitano en Salud Mental. *Anales de Salud Mental*, Vol. XVIII. 2002; 135–46.
3. Instituto Nacional de Salud Mental "Honorio Delgado - Hideyo Noguchi". Estudio Epidemiológico Metropolitano en Salud Mental en la Sierra Peruana. *Anales de Salud Mental*, Vol. XIX. 2003; 143–60.
4. Ganguli M, Ratcliff G, Huff F, *et al.* Effect of age, gender, and education on cognitive tests in a rural elderly community sample: Norms from the Monongahela Valley Independent Elders Survey. *Neuroepidemiology* 1991; **10**: 42–52.

Chapter

9B The clinical approach to the person with dementia

Nigeria

Richard Uwakwe

Presentation

A patient with dementia (in Nigeria) will most often be brought for medical attention by family members. More often than not the accompanying family member is the spouse, although children and daughters-/sons-in-law etc. may accompany the individual on occasion. At the time of presentation the most likely reason for seeking medical attention will be the behavioral and psychological symptoms of dementia (BPSD), rather than memory or other cognitive features. When memory problems are predominant, especially at the early stages, normal aging rather than disease is often mistakenly thought to be the cause. Indeed, many primary care physicians would concur with the notion that memory problems in the elderly are "senile dementia" (wrongly) attributed to be part of normal aging. This delays presentation for clinical attention to specialists like neurologists or psychiatrics.

The history given is often poor and lacking in detail and the clinician is expected to diagnose the patient's problem, once the informants state that the person is behaving inappropriately. Detailed questions are often seen as being embarrassing, irrelevant, and unrelated to the patient's problem. A combination of finely honed clinical skills and intimate knowledge of indigenous sociocultural norms are therefore required to elicit informative and useful clinical history. Often times, insomnia, wandering, getting lost, and displaying socially embarrassing behavior are the factors most burdensome to the family.

Pathway

It is near impossible for the psychiatrist, neurologist, or other medical officer to be the first person who is consulted. In nearly every case the patient would have been taken to alternative medical treatment centers including churches, native healing homes, etc. A diagnosis of poisoning, wicked spirits, "ndiotu" (that is special spiritual peer groups) would have been made in these alternative centers.

Dementia: A Global Approach, ed. Ennapadam S. Krishnamoorthy, Martin J. Prince, and Jeffrey L. Cummings. Published by Cambridge University Press.

Examination and investigation

Following information gathering, a mental state examination is conducted. Elaborate neuropsychological tests are often not done. In any case the stage of dementia is most likely to be moderate to severe (it is rare to see early or mild stages/phases). Physical, including neurological, examination is conducted. Laboratory investigations are often few and cover only basic parameters. Family members expect diagnosis from the physician there and then, and it is unacceptable to postpone diagnosis even for a day. This fact, including limitation of fund and facilities, often means that complex investigations are not done – including CT, MRI, B12, folate, thyroid function studies, etc. Only in certain (generally rare) instances where it is clinically indicated are these investigations carried out. In most cases the diagnosis is achieved on purely clinical grounds.

Management

Conveying the diagnosis poses a particular challenge for clinicians in Nigeria, as in most cases Nigerians expect miraculous, instantaneous, and permanent cure. Psychological treatments including behavioral modifications or group support are not generally appreciated; instead the common desire is for a magic drug that will cure, preferably one strong injection. While the physician may in all likelihood prescribe cognitive enhancers and appropriate psychotropic medications, their effects are often seen as disappointing. For example, donepezil is now available in Nigeria (though extremely costly by Nigerian standard) but in spite of what the physician may discuss with caregivers, they are likely to return within three days to report that the client is still behaving the same way. Inappropriate use of psychotropics and hypnotics often produces unacceptable drowsiness and other side effects. Use of medication has to be therefore extremely cautious as the side effects may result in patients and families dropping out of follow-up. The physician in this setting will find it useful to discuss with the entire family: the implications of diagnosis; the possible need for long-term care; and the importance and utility of sharing care activities within the family. In some instances, it is recommended that the patient be cared for in a rotational manner among the daughters or daughters-in-law. Dementia nursing homes or other such facilities are not available in Nigeria. A lot of the times this arrangement of shared care by female family members (while men are encouraged to contribute financial and other material needs) may sustain the client for a reasonable length of time. State aids or health insurance and other social security measures are not available; families are entirely responsible for the overall care of their elderly relation who has dementia. In instances where the patient who has dementia does not have children or other close family relations, community social groups are mobilized to assist. In some instances the church or group within the organization accepts to take the responsibility to care for the patient. Many Nigerian families are often large with extended kinship and this sometimes serves as a safety valve. Caregivers often feel very burdened with the patient's disability, incontinence (bladder or bowel or both) being especially stressful to the caregiver, as modern toilet facilities with running water are oftentimes not available with pit latrines and the habit of squatting in the shrub continuing to be commonplace in many communities. Many Nigerian elderly are not used to Western-style closets. In this cultural context clinical advice to the caregiver includes the constant checking and changing of mats or beddings; restricted fluid intake towards bedtime; and bladder and bowel emptying at regular intervals, all of which minimize episodes of incontinence. In some instances we make use of Paul's tubing for males and continence pads (such as are used in infants) for females.

Comorbid medical diseases like hypertension, other cardiovascular problems, type 2 diabetes mellitus, arthritis, etc. are managed accordingly. Dropout rate is enormous and the patient may be taken to other medical or alternative treatments in an attempt to get the desired permanent cure – an expensive exercise!

Nutrition

Carbohydrate products are often the staple food in Nigeria. Vitamins and other supplements may be given. When swallowing becomes difficult at the late stages of dementia, feeding can become problematic. Nasogastric tube and central parenteral feeding are difficult to practice, especially outside the orthodox hospital setting. Feeding is encouraged in fluid form in small doses.

Legal issues

It is unusual for a patient with dementia to have had a driving license, prior to the development of dementia. Loss of driving license is therefore rarely a problem. Most Nigerians do not make wills before death; testamentary capacity, appointment of power of attorney, etc. are therefore rare issues in the culture. The tradition seems to have an "in-built will" in operation, starting with the first male child. What is more likely is loss of privilege or position of responsibility in social groups (churches, unions, other associations, etc.) which hardly has any legal implications.

End-of-life issues

Facilities for long-term sustenance in assisted living are rare. It is not usual to be faced with the difficulties of keeping alive a patient who is seen as a vegetable. Prior medical directives as to the patient's wishes in such instances will almost always be absent.

Postmortem studies

For both cultural and religious reasons most Nigerian families would not permit a postmortem examination. Death of the elderly is preferred to occur at home and elaborate funeral rites are performed. The histological diagnosis of Alzheimer's disease is therefore not achieved in most cases, with diagnosis and management being based on a high index of clinical suspicion in our setting.

The clinical approach to the person with dementia

Australia

David Ames and Eleanor Flynn

Introduction

The approach to the detection, assessment, diagnosis, and management of an Australian dementia patient is colored by geography (the challenge of distance), demography (a rapidly aging and increasingly ethnically diverse population), the structure and funding of the Australian health system, and the availability of specific services for people with dementia.

Geography, demography, and government structure

Australia is a nation of 22 million people, occupying a landmass similar in size to the continental United States. Although there are several remote and rural communities, most of Australia's population is clustered in coastal cities. Thirteen percent of Australians are aged 65 and above and that proportion is growing rapidly. A quarter of those aged over 65 were born outside Australia and for one in four of the overseas-born elderly, English is not their mother tongue [1]. Aboriginals and Torres Strait islanders comprise 1% of the elderly population. Many of them live in remote areas and their particular cultural and economic situations require a different pattern of dementia service delivery than that offered to urban Anglo-Celts [2]. The national government collects the bulk of taxation revenue and passes some of it to the six state and two territory governments, who are charged with the delivery of hospital care [1].

Health and aged care services in Australia

Although hospital and some community psychiatric care is delivered by state governments, the national government funds Medicare, a universal health insurance scheme, which pays most of the cost of ambulatory consultations with primary care physicians (general practitioners) and medical specialists, and some of the cost of medical consultations and procedures in private hospitals, for which somewhat less than one-third of Australians carry additional commercially sourced insurance.

Dementia: A Global Approach, ed. Ennapadam S. Krishnamoorthy, Martin J. Prince, and Jeffrey L. Cummings. Published by Cambridge University Press.

All regions of Australia are covered by over 100 geriatrician-led Aged Care Assessment teams (ACATs) [3], whose main function is to assess individuals who may need to enter permanent residential care. It is common for ACATs to arrange services to support aged individuals so that they can remain in the community. Some support services are funded by the Health and Community Care (HACC) scheme and vary from the simple provision of meals, or home help, to a full aged care package delivering many hours per week of specialized assistance.

A consultation with a medical specialist will not attract a Medicare rebate unless the patient has been referred by a primary care physician. A small but growing number of psychiatrists, geriatricians, and neurologists have a specific interest in dementia and will assess referred patients who are thought to be affected by early dementia symptoms. The state of Victoria has several state government-funded Cognitive Assessment and Dementia Management Services (CADMS). These are memory clinics, staffed by medical specialists, nurses, and allied health staff, including a neuropsychologist, but in other states the availability of memory clinic services is patchy and their funding arrangements tend to be ad hoc [1]. Victoria also has the best-developed psychiatric provision for elderly people and provides dedicated aged psychiatry inpatient and community services (see below).

Detection, assessment, and diagnosis

Detection of dementia continues to be a major challenge, particularly among the very old. Increased community awareness of the availability of treatment and services for dementia has led to earlier presentation, but it is still common for cases to present at an advanced stage of cognitive decline.

Assessment by most primary care physicians tends to be brief, because the current system of primary care physician remuneration rewards multiple short consultations more generously than a few long ones. However, recent funding changes now pay primary care physicians well for attendance at multidisciplinary case meetings for patients over the age of 75 years.

Simple cognitive screening tools such as the Mini-Mental State Examination (MMSE) [4] are commonly used by primary care physicians, but most would refer a patient suspected of having an early dementia to a private specialist or a CADMS/memory clinic [5,6] for further assessment. In the specialist setting, great emphasis would be placed on eliciting a reliable informant history, which is crucial to the accurate assessment of dementia. After the taking of a history and performance of a mental state examination, in addition to the MMSE most specialists would either undertake a more detailed cognitive assessment such as the ADAS-Cog [7] or CAMCOG [8] or refer the patient to a neuropsychologist. A full physical examination forms an integral part of dementia assessment in most specialist settings. Neuropsychologists are available in most memory clinics and an increasing number are available in urban areas to assess privately referred patients.

Most suspected dementia patients undergo cerebral imaging with CT or MRI. A typical blood screen would consist of full blood exam, erythrocyte sedimentation rate, B12 and folate, thyroid-stimulating hormone (TSH), urea, creatinine and electrolytes, liver function tests, glucose, lipid profile, calcium, phosphate, and (less often) syphilis serology. Most non-smokers would not undergo chest X-ray [6].

A major focus of specialist assessment for dementia in Australia is on reaching a definite diagnosis. Does the patient exhibit a dementia syndrome as defined in the International Classification of Diseases, tenth edition (ICD-10) [9], or is he/she affected by mild cognitive impairment, depression, "normal aging," or is he/she in fact cognitively intact? If a dementia is present is it due to Alzheimer's disease (AD) (the NINCDS-ADRDA criteria [10] are widely employed in teaching settings), is there a vascular component, or does the patient have frontotemporal dementia, dementia with Lewy bodies, or some rarer condition?

Once a diagnosis has been reached, a key responsibility is to give information about the diagnosis, likely prognosis, and planned management to the patient, supported by key family members [5].

Management of cognitive impairment in dementia

The majority of AD patients diagnosed by specialists in Australia are offered a trial of treatment with a cholinesterase inhibitor. Donepezil, rivastigmine, and galantamine are all available and subsidized by the prescriber benefit scheme at a direct cost to pensioners of $A4.90 ($A1 = $US0.83, £0.57 and €0.67 in May 2010) per prescription ($30.70 to non-pensioners), but the rules covering their prescription are cumbersome. Patients must be diagnosed as having AD by a consultant physician (internal medicine specialist) or psychiatrist (a primary care physician diagnosis is insufficient), must have a baseline MMSE or ADAS-Cog score recorded (the former must be 10 or greater to qualify for treatment), and a written application for treatment (which takes up to two weeks to process) must be submitted. Patients may only receive further prescriptions after six months of therapy if they demonstrate a minimum 2-point improvement in MMSE score or a 4-point ADAS-Cog benefit. For patients who are illiterate, cannot speak the language of the examiner, or who for cultural reasons cannot complete the MMSE or ADAS-Cog, it is permitted for the prescribing specialist to perform a Clinician-Based Impression of Change assessment which documents improvement on therapy.

Memantine is available, but is little used because it is unsubsidized and costs patients $A120 per month. Vitamin E never enjoyed in Australia the popularity it attained for the treatment of AD in the USA, and following new concerns about safety [11] it is now little used. Australia has been and continues to be a significant contributor of patient numbers to multicenter international trials of new pharmacological agents to treat dementia [12].

Alzheimer's Australia runs excellent information, education, and support services, but not every newly diagnosed patient is referred for this assistance, and only some of those who are referred actually attend.

Management of behavioral and psychological symptoms of dementia (BPSD)

In the state of Victoria the state government funds catchment area-based Aged Psychiatry Assessment and Treatment teams (APATTs), which cover the entire state. The service formerly led by the first author is responsible for a population of 45 000 people aged 65 and above and conducts about 700 new community assessments annually, as well as running a 20-bed inpatient unit and 60 psychogeriatric nursing home beds. The largest diagnostic group served by these teams consists of individuals affected by BPSD. A large component of this work consists in educating family and professional carers about the nature and management of BPSD. Advice about prescription of psychotropic drugs is made under the direction of a consultant psychiatrist attached to the APATT. In other states, public aged psychiatry services are less well developed, though most capital cities have consultant-led community aged psychiatry services free at the point of delivery. Psychotropic drugs are used liberally by primary care physicians to treat dementia patients in nursing homes, despite concerns about safety and questionable efficacy [13].

The care of the patient with advanced dementia

Around 7% of elderly Australians live in nursing homes or hostels, where their care is heavily subsidized by the national government. The majority of these residents have dementia and at least half of all Australians with moderate to severe dementia live in residential care.

References

1. LoGiudice D, Flynn E, Ames D. Services to people with dementia: a worldwide view – Australia. In: Burns A, O'Brien J, Ames D, eds. *Dementia*, 3rd edn. London, Hodder Arnold. 2005; 256–60.
2. LoGiudice D, Smith K, Thomas J, *et al.* Kimberly Indigenous Cognitive Assessment tool (KICA): development of a cognitive assessment tool for older indigenous Australians. *Int Psychogeriatr* 2006; **18**: 269–80.
3. Howe A. From states of confusion to a National Action Plan for Dementia Care. *Int J Geriatr Psychiatry* 1997; **12**: 165–71.
4. Folstein MF, Folstein SE, McHugh PR. Mini-mental state: a practical method for grading the cognitive state of patients for the clinician. *J Psychiatr Res* 1975; **12**: 189–98.
5. Ames D, Flicker L, Helme R. A memory clinic at a geriatric hospital: rationale, routine and review of the first 100 patients. *Med J Aust* 1992; **156**: 618–22.
6. Stratford JA, Logiudice D, Flicker L, *et al.* A memory clinic at a geriatric hospital: a report on 577 patients assessed with the CAMDEX over 9 years. *Aust N Z J Psychiatry*, 2003; **37**: 319–26.
7. Rosen WG, Mohs RC, Davis KL. A new rating scale for Alzheimer's disease. *Am J Psychiatry* 1984; **141**: 1356–64.
8. Roth M, Tym E, Mountjoy CQ, *et al.* CAMDEX: a standardized instrument for the diagnosis of mental disorder in the elderly with special reference to the early detection of dementia. *Br J Psychiatry* 1986; **149**: 698–709.
9. World Health Organization. *The ICD-10 Classification of Mental and Behavioural Disorders. Diagnostic Criteria for Research.* Geneva, World Health Organization, 1993.
10. McKhann G, Drachman D, Folstein M, *et al.* Clinical diagnosis of Alzheimer's disease. Report of the NINCDS-ADRDA work group under the auspices of the Department of Health and

Human Services Task Force on Alzheimer's disease. *Neurology* 1984; **34**: 939–44.

11. Ames D, Ritchie C. Antioxidants and Alzheimer's disease: time to stop feeding vitamin E to dementia patients? *Int Psychogeriatr* 2007; **19**: 1–8.
12. Ames D. Geriatric psychiatry in Australia. *Int J Geriatr Psychiatry* 1997; **12**: 143–4.
13. Ames D, Ballard C, Cream J, *et al.* For debate: should novel antipsychotics ever be used to treat the behavioral and psychological symptoms of dementia (BPSD)? *Int Psychogeriatr* 2005; **17**: 3–29.

The clinical approach to the person with dementia

The United States of America

Jeffrey L. Cummings

Introduction

Dementia care in the USA has the following characteristics: (1) the number of patients with dementia is anticipated to increase; (2) most patients in private practice are not diagnosed until late in the clinical course when dementia is of moderate severity; (3) most patients with dementia have part of the cost of care borne by Medicare and Medicaid, the national health insurance policies for the elderly; (4) academic care of dementia patients tends to use advanced diagnostic technology and combination regimens of pharmacological agents; and (5) disease-modifying therapy is anticipated and is likely to reshape dementia care in the USA.

The number of patients with dementia will increase

The number of people over the age of 65 in the USA is expected to double from approximately 35 million in 2007 to more than 70 million by 2030 [1]. Dementia is an age-related disorder and the increased number of elderly individuals inevitably implies that there will be a greater number of dementia patients over time. Current estimates of the prevalence of dementia vary; a recent study indicated a prevalence of 3 407 000 (range 2 793 000 to 4 021 000) [1]. Of these 70% had Alzheimer's disease (AD) and 17% had vascular dementia (VaD). The relative frequency of AD increased with age, so that in the 90-plus-year-old age group AD accounted for 80% of dementia cases. The overall prevalence of dementia increased with age from affecting approximately 5% of those age 71 to 79 to 37% of those age 90 and older. A recent study by the Alzheimer's Association [2] places the total number of AD victims at 5.1 million rising from 2% in those aged 65 to 74, to 19% among individuals 75 to 84, and to 42% in those of 85 and older. The number of annual new cases is expected to rise from 454 000 in 2010 to 615 000 by the year 2030 and to 959 000 new cases a year by 2050, unless some means of

Dementia: A Global Approach, ed. Ennapadam S. Krishnamoorthy, Martin J. Prince, and Jeffrey L. Cummings. Published by Cambridge University Press.

preventing or delaying the onset of AD is discovered and effectively implemented.

The increasing size of the dementia population and the tremendous cost imposed by dementia care will require substantial reorganization of services to meet this expanding public health need.

Dementia is under-recognized

Despite the known high prevalence of dementia among the elderly, many patients with cognitive impairment do not receive a diagnosis of AD or other dementia syndrome, or diagnosis is delayed until late in the clinical course. Studies place the rate of recognition at between 20% and 30% with 70% to 80% of patients going unrecognized early in the clinical course [3,4].

A variety of circumstances contribute to the low rate of recognition and diagnosis of dementia. Among those cited by primary care physicians include insufficient time, difficulty accessing and communicating with specialists, low reimbursements for dementia care, poor communication with social service agencies, and lack of interdisciplinary teams with relevant expertise [5].

Even among patients who receive a diagnosis of dementia or AD, the rate of therapeutic intervention is low. Sano and colleagues [6] found that among patients recruited for a trial of anti-dementia therapy, only 65% had previously been treated with such agents. This rate is likely higher than in general practice settings.

Preliminary steps have been taken to determine whether compliance with diagnosis and treatment guidelines can be enhanced in a randomized trial of a disease management program. Adherence was significantly better in the intervention group when compared with the no-intervention group (64% compared to 33%) [7].This suggests that practitioners and healthcare systems can be influenced to adhere to treatment guidelines with educational interventions.

Medicare and Medicaid fund most direct care costs of dementia care

It is estimated that in 2005 the cost for caring for demented patients in the USA was approximately 100 billion dollars; this is expected to reach 1 trillion dollars by 2050 [3]. Such costs are likely to exceed the resources available through Medicare and other public health funding.

The cost of anti-dementia medications to Medicaid has been analyzed. Morden *et al.* [8] found that 4.4% of Medicaid beneficiaries received anti-dementia medications; projecting this figures to 2006 resulted in an annual estimated cost of 990 million dollars annually. This represents 3% of 32 billion cost of Medicaid pharmaceutical expenditures.

Behavioral disturbances are common in AD and other dementia syndromes and patients with behavioral disturbances have greater associated costs than those without [9].

Academic medical centers rely on advanced technology and combined treatment regimens

Academic medical centers in the USA are at the cutting edge of AD care. There is a rapid technology transfer of new diagnostic strategies with many patients evaluated with magnetic resonance imaging (MRI) and fluorodeoxy glucose positron emission tomography (FDG-PET). It is anticipated that amyloid PET will be available soon, making molecular imaging routinely available to clinicians. The widespread availability of tests with higher diagnostic specificity may tend to increase the rate of diagnosis and therapy.

Physicians practicing in academic medical centers also tend to implement more complete therapeutic regimens readily. Combined treatment with cholinesterase and memantine is common and it is anticipated that disease-modifying therapies (discussed below) will be integrated into therapeutic regimens.

Disease-modifying agents may reshape dementia care in the USA

Improved understanding of the molecular mechanisms of AD has led to the identification of several exploitable pharmacological targets. Success in modulating these pathways is anticipated to produce disease modification with slowing of disease progression. Successful introduction of disease-modifying treatments into the market and the therapeutic armamentarium is likely to have profound effects.

The advent of disease-modifying treatments may motivate many more practitioners to identify patients with AD and to attempt to identify them earlier in the disease course when introduction of disease-modifying therapies will have the greatest impact. More aggressive diagnosis will result in a greater number of identified patients in the healthcare system requesting services. Treatment will be initiated with the attendant costs of the compound and care of any side effects. Monitoring of therapy will require follow-up assessments. The need for laboratory studies will depend on the side effect and safety profile of the treatment.

Attempts at early diagnosis by less experienced practitioners will result in more false positive diagnoses and a need to "un-diagnose" more patients by specialists.

Biomarkers assist in identifying patients with the early form of AD [10] and MRI, FDG-PET, amyloid PET, or studies of amyloid and tau protein in cerebrospinal fluid will be performed more often.

Agents that slow progression will result in deferring major milestones of AD such as decline to greater levels of dependency, emergence of behavioral abnormalities, and nursing home placement. Survival may be prolonged if death does not occur through competitive mortality of the aged. This outcome will have marked influence on health care economics in the USA.

It is currently uncertain if disease-modifying agents will increase or decrease the cost of care. If they slow progression and defer nursing home placement without prolonging survival and the duration of nursing home care, they will likely decrease the cost of care. If they increase disease duration and prolong the period of nursing home care, they will most likely increase the cost of the care of dementia patients.

Dementia care in the USA will thus in all likelihood be reshaped by emerging therapies and new technologies.

Acknowledgments

Dr. Cummings is supported by a National Institute on Aging Alzheimer's Disease Research

Center grant (P50 AG16570), an Alzheimer's Research Center of California grant, the Sidell Kagan Foundation, Mary S. Easton Gift and the Deane F. Johnson Alzheimer's Research Foundation.

References

1. Plassman PL, Langa KM, Fisher GG, *et al.* Prevalence of dementia in the United States: The Aging, Demographics, and Memory Study. *Neuroepidemiology* 2007; **29**:125–32.
2. Alzheimer's Association. *Alzheimer's Disease Facts and Figures 2007.* Washington, DC, Alzheimer's Association, 2007.
3. Brayne C, Fox C, Boustani M. Dementia screening in primary care – Is it time? *JAMA* 2007; **298**: 2409–11.
4. Boustani M, Callahan CM, Unverzagt FW, *et al.* Implementing a screening and diagnosis program for dementia in primary care. *J Gen Intern Med* 2005; **20**: 572–7.
5. Hinton L, Franz C, Reddy G, *et al.* Practice constraints, behavioral problems, and dementia care: primary care physicians' perspectives. *J Gen Intern Med* 2007; **22**: 1487–92.
6. Sano M, Amatniek J, Feely M, *et al.* Undertreatment of patients with Alzheimer's disease in an elderly United States population. *Alzheimer's Dement* 2005; **1**:136–144.
7. Vickery B, Mittman B, Connor K, *et al.* The effect of a disease management intervention on quality and outcomes of dementia care. *Ann Intern Med* 2006; **145**: 713–26.
8. Morden N, Zerzan J, Larson EB. Alzheimer's disease dedication: use and cost projections for Medicare Part D. *J Am Geriatr Assoc* 2007; **55**: 622–4.
9. Murman DL, Chen Q, Powell MC, *et al.* The incremental direct costs associated with behavioral symptoms in AD. *Neurology* 2002; **59**: 1721–9.
10. Dubois B, Jacova J, DeKosky J, *et al.* Research criteria for the diagnosis of Alzheimer's disease: revising the NINCDS–ADRDA criteria. *Lancet Neurol* 2007; **6**: 734–46.

Chapter

9E

The clinical approach to the person with dementia

Japan

Akira Homma

Introduction

The changes to the Japanese long-term care insurance that came into force in April 2000, such as the switch from measures and plans to actual contracts; the guarantee of selection and rights; and the offer of unified health, medical, and welfare services, marked a major turning point in the history of nursing care for the elderly in Japan. Also, the first review of the insurance fees and premiums, as well as revision of the compensation paid to caregivers, was conducted in April 2003. In March 2003 the "Elderly Care Study Group" was established in response to a request from the Health and Welfare Bureau for the Elderly, of the Japanese Ministry of Health, Labor, and Welfare. The purpose was to identify problems and issues concerning care of the elderly, under the long-term care insurance, and to study how to deal from then on with these issues of care for the elderly and the social systems needed to support such care. Put more simply, the objective of the Elderly Care Study Group is to put forth proposals concerning the direction of a new plan to succeed the Gold Plan 21 aiming the direction of health and welfare policies for the elderly from 2000 to 2004. The study group has met and held hearings with experts, a total of ten times, and issued a report dealing with nursing care for the elderly in 2015. This report was compiled keeping in mind the need to implement this plan by 2015, the year in which the tail end of the postwar Japanese baby-boom generation will become 65 years old, an event of significance for Japan. In the report, it states that even if an elderly person is in a condition that requires nursing care, it is possible for the person to live as he/she wishes, and that one important aim is the realization of care that maintains the dignity of the elderly. The report also touches upon the discussion regarding making the nursing care system a sustainable entity.

Present situation concerning nursing care for the elderly following implementation of the long-term care insurance

The most significant change is the increase in the number of people using nursing care

Dementia: A Global Approach, ed. Ennapadam S. Krishnamoorthy, Martin J. Prince, and Jeffrey L. Cummings. Published by Cambridge University Press.

services, especially the number of people using in-home nursing care services, which has doubled [1]. The number of companies providing nursing care services for the elderly has also increased by an average of 11.4% [1]. While the rate of increase in the number of users has surpassed the rate of increase in the number of companies, it does appear, based on the numbers anyway, that the system for providing nursing care services is in the process of becoming established. Comparison of the persons requesting nursing care in 1996 and 2002, in other words, before and after implementation of the long-term care insurance, reveals that while there was no change in the proportion of caregiving being requested for spouses (53%), there were relatively large decreases in the percentages for a child and the spouse of a child, from 71% to 53% and 38% to 25%, respectively [2]. There may be a possibility that a part of the care provided by a child or the spouse of a child is replaced by the services of the long-term care insurance. Thus, the influence of service use through the long-term care insurance cannot be denied.

The second point is that the number of people officially designated as requiring nursing care has increased at a greater pace than the actual increase in the number of elderly people [1]. The increase in the number of mild cases (those designated as requiring assistance and Level 1 care) has been particularly remarkable. This suggests that it has become possible to use the services beginning at an earlier stage compared to the past. However, it is possible that other factors, besides those related to the expanded use of the system, are involved, if we take into consideration the large variation between regions in the percentage of persons who require assistance and those who require Level 1 nursing care compared to Level 4 and 5 nursing care.

The third point, if we examine the changes in the care needs assessment results, is that the percentage improvement in the degree of care required is less for mild cases compared to more severely affected persons who are rated as Level 2 or above. If we consider the definition of "requiring assistance," which is "there is concern that the person is in a state that may require nursing care," it is conceivable that care prevention/intervention was not efficiently provided to mild cases in whom the effect of any prevention/intervention could be more or less expected. This kind of trend suggests that a reexamination of ideal care prevention/intervention activities and rehabilitation is needed.

One of the objectives of the long-term care insurance is to maintain the lives of the elderly at home. As mentioned above, this corresponds to the increase in the use of home services. However, on the other hand, it has also been pointed out that there is a dramatic increase in the number of people applying for nursing homes for the elderly. Under the long-term care insurance, eligible persons are free to apply for admission to these facilities. However, some elderly who do not need to enter such a facility right away are applying in advance, creating a sort of reservation or waiting-list type of situation. According to the results of a survey conducted by a health insurance union, only an approximate 30% of the people who are applying are actually thought by the staff to require admission, meaning that over 60% of the applicants are still able to live at home by themselves. However, a survey conducted by the Office of the Cabinet found that

60% of elderly people, who need nursing care, expressed a desire to live at home. Examination of the use of nursing care services shows that less than half of the people requiring a high degree of nursing care are living at home, indicating that at the present level, services cannot provide support for all those needing care, to live in their own home [1]. If we look at where the elderly are dying, it can be seen that in recent years almost 80% are passing away at a medical facility. However, approximately half of the people responding to the question "if you develop an incurable disease, where would you like to spend your last days?" answered their own home. This demonstrates all too clearly that the present situation is one in which the elderly do not necessarily die where they wish (see also Chapter 9B on Nigeria).

The fourth point is the increase in individualized care, such as unit care, fee-charging nursing homes with care and apartment houses with care services. Since 2002, the Japanese government has been making financial support available for maintenance and upkeep of facilities that provide unit care. Individual care, even at a facility where group care is the norm, has been increasing. The number of group homes for dementia persons has increased from 30 in 1998 to about 900 in 2001, an increase of 30-fold, and to an astonishing 6800 in 2004 (more than a 200-fold increase compared to 1998). Since group homes are considered to be an in-home service, they account for a mere 2–3% of all in-home services. While it is unmistakable that the individual care system has commenced, it is not yet in a position in which its benefits be evaluated fully, because, like nursing homes for the elderly, access to this form of care is limited to certain individuals and is not available therefore for general use. Furthermore, the differences in outcome between nursing homes for the elderly and unit care or group homes have not been subject to scientific scrutiny. If the quality of life of the elderly person with dementia can be evaluated in these different settings, differences between these three service delivery models may emerge and these data are urgently required in order to determine what constitutes best care for dementia in Japan.

The fifth point is the fact that dementia has been confirmed in more than half of all eligible people requiring nursing care [1] This means there are three issues. The first is a result of the original long-term care insurance. That is, even though the stress experienced by care providers caring for bedridden elderly not thought to have dementia was alleviated following the introduction of the long-term care insurance, the burden of caregivers looking after able-bodied elderly with dementia increased [3]. While this has been demonstrated only by one local government, it was obtained before and after the introduction of the long-term care insurance, and assumes great significance given that these data cannot be obtained again, long-term insurance having been implemented widely. The second issue, which is already well known, is that approximately 70% of dementia-related disorders in late life are treated medically. It is significant that Alzheimer's disease, the underlying disease which accounts for the large proportion of dementia seen in old age, is now treated with medication.

Even though half of all elderly, officially designated as requiring nursing care, have dementia, it is not clear what percentage of these people have actually received a proper medical diagnosis. What appears certain is that a diagnosis of "dementia" has been clearly stated by the physician on the patient's chart in all these cases. However, the clear identification of subtypes such as Alzheimer-type dementia or vascular dementia is rare.

Self-report cases (people who check themselves in to the medical facility with the suspicion of dementia) are extremely rare in the Japanese context and the lack of knowledge and recognition of dementia by the family and in many instances the primary healthcare professional remains a barrier for early diagnosis. While we will not delve into the details here, it goes without saying, that a person has the right to receive appropriate medical treatment, if he/she sick, even if is unable to visit a physician or hospital on his/her own. The failure to provide such care may be construed as amounting to neglect by the family or health professional, by ignoring the rights of the elderly person. To put it another way, the examination, diagnosis, and treatment of an elderly person with dementia needing a mild degree of assistance or nursing care (i.e., Level 1) early on assumes significance from the point of view of preventing the need for nursing care. The third issue is that the adult guardianship system, which was started simultaneously with nursing care insurance, is not functioning to protect the rights of elderly dementia persons with impaired mental capacity. The major deficiency of the adult guardianship system is that it is not clear who has the authority to give medical consent. For this reason, it was reported in Japanese newspapers in 2003 and 2004 that some elderly did not receive influenza vaccination even though their guardians had been designated. Because one out of two elderly people officially designated as requiring nursing care has some sort of impairment to their mental capacity, it is not an exaggeration to say that there is currently no workable system in Japan for these people to receive appropriate medical treatment and whether their premorbid lifestyle and dignity can be maintained under these circumstances is questionable.

Policies and measures for the establishment of nursing care that maintains dignity

A conceptual representation of policies and measures for the establishment of care that maintains dignity based on the types of issues and concerns comprises (1) establishment of a new care model: dementia care, (2) a new nursing care service system that maintains the lifestyle in place before nursing care becomes necessary, (3) ensuring and improving the quality of service and (4) rehabilitation and preventing the need for nursing care. These four points are all interrelated. Also, while it is correct to say that a variety of issues surrounding nursing care for the elderly has come to light, during implementation of the long-term care insurance system, not all four points described here will be solved by the nursing care insurance system. The background surrounding the establishment of these four pillars has been dealt with previously together with the issues arising after implementation of the long-term care insurance; however, a few things should be added.

With respect to ensuring and improving the quality of service, care managers who are responsible for constructing care plans should understand care management while at the same time being skilled in the assessment and care management plan development for elderly persons with dementia. At present, care managers do not appear to consider family problems surrounding the elderly person designated as needing nursing care as part of their job. Also, the present situation is that not all care managers recognize that dementia is an obvious disease, or that Alzheimer-type dementia can be treated medically. The Dementia Care Research and Training Centers located in three areas of Japan have produced guidelines that are suitable for persons with dementia and the model projects conducted in 2004 at 16 locations throughout Japan have revealed the utility of these guidelines in improving the quality of care. Although there are many areas of weakness in the local services alluded to previously with respect to the establishment of standardization and methodology of care, we must simultaneously think about a system in local areas for the discovery of dementia at an early phase. Such studies are currently in progress. In the same way, based on the results from model training projects in 16 locations throughout Japan with an aim to improve the diagnostic techniques for dementia of family physicians, in cooperation with the Japan Medical Association from 2004 to 2005, and the Ministry of Health, Labor, and Welfare we (the author and colleagues) commenced nationwide in 2006 a training and education program for family physicians. The number of the primary care physicians who participated in the program was 21 444 from 2006 to 2008. Furthermore, new service delivery systems with the lifestyle maintenance mandate have significant meaning in terms of care for elderly patients with dementia. While a variety of services are presently being offered, such as "trips to and from a hospital," "overnight stay at a facility," "receiving home visits," and "living at a facility," many problems and issues may be solved if the same professional caregiver (staff member) is in charge of the patient through the process. Whether it is unit care or a group home, in many cases the elderly person is forced to leave the home they have become accustomed to, and become separated from friends and loved-ones. There are therefore numerous problems that need to be resolved. Additional issues that must be dealt with include the construction of small-scale, multifunction facilities in large cities; quality assurance; sustainable methods of cooperation with medical institutions; and the limits to which long-term care insurance can pay for such care. These unresolved issues notwithstanding, individual or person-centered care based on the person's premorbid lifestyle needs to become part of active care models for dementia in Japan and world over.

References

1. MHLW. *Elderly Care Study Group Report, Elderly Care in 2015 – Toward the Establishment of a Care Service System to Support the Dignity of Elderly People*. General Affairs Division, Health and Welfare Bureau for the Elderly, the Ministry of Health, Labour, and Welfare, June, 2003.
2. The Office of the Cabinet. *The Survey Report of the Recognition of Health of the Elderly*, May, 2003.
3. Niina R, Homma A. Change of the stress responses of in-home caregivers before and after the introduction of the long-term-care insurance in Machida city. *Jpn J Geriatr Psychiatry* 2002; **13**: 517–523.

Chapter

9F The clinical approach to the person with dementia

China

Joshua Tsoh, Helen Chiu, and Xin Yu

Introduction

China has 32 provinces and 2 special administrative regions (Hong Kong and Macau) and at least 57 ethnic groups with vast diversity in their cultures, traditions, dialects, and attitudes towards medical illnesses, including dementia. There is also significant heterogeneity in local socioeconomic states and medical infrastructures. Hence, there is no unified approach to dementia care within the nation. We will start by outlining the known practices in Hong Kong and in the urban and rural areas of mainland China, and highlight the differences.

Approach to patients with dementia I: the Special Administrative Region of Hong Kong

Hong Kong is arguably the most "Westernized" city in China through its colonial legacy (please refer to Chapter 7C on care arrangements for patients with dementia in China). With a medical infrastructure and training curriculum that is modeled on the British system, the regular clinical approaches/protocols for the assessment and clinical management of dementia are not significantly different from those in Western countries.

In Hong Kong, patients with dementia most commonly present to primary care and upon recognition of the syndrome are referred to psychiatrists or geriatricians for further assessment and management. Detailed history taking, a complete physical, mental, and cognitive state examination and investigations including blood tests and radiological examinations of the brain are performed for accurate diagnosis and subtyping of dementia. Assessment instruments like the Mini-Mental State Examination (MMSE) are frequently used.

Clinical diagnosis is usually based on the International Classification of Diseases, tenth edition (ICD-10) [1] or Diagnostic and Statistical Manual of Mental Disorders, fourth edition (DSM-IV) [2] criteria. As part of psychogeriatric

Dementia: A Global Approach, ed. Ennapadam S. Krishnamoorthy, Martin J. Prince, and Jeffrey L. Cummings. Published by Cambridge University Press.

teams, occupational therapists and physiotherapists are involved in the assessment of the functional and physical deficits associated with dementia. Community psychiatric nurses and social workers investigate the social and home conditions for patients' service needs, safety for community living, and the degree of caregiver support and coping. In indicated cases, a speech therapist's assessment of the swallowing function, not uncommonly disturbed in dementia, is arranged.

Treatment of dementia is likewise multidisciplinary. Guidelines for drug treatment in public services are laid down by the Psychogeriatric Working Group in Hong Kong; they are similar to those promulgated by the National Institute for Health and Clinical Excellence (NICE) in the UK or the American Psychiatric Association (APA) in the USA. In indicated cases (e.g., early or moderate Alzheimer's disease [AD], or dementia with Lewy bodies), acetylcholinesterase inhibitors (AChEIs) are prescribed. The usual choices include donepezil, rivastigmine, and galatamine. Cognitive function is monitored periodically (e.g., quarterly). For patients with moderate or severe AD, glutamate antagonists like memantine may be prescribed. Vitamin E has fallen out of favor as a treatment for AD following recent meta-analyses, showing its lack of efficacy and slightly increased mortality rates associated with high dosage [3]. For cases with behavioral and psychological symptoms of dementia (BPSD), non-pharmacological strategies, including behavioral analyses and therapies, and measures to optimize the level of sensory stimuli in the environment are the first line of interventions. For severe cases, psychotropic drugs including antipsychotics, antidepressants, and anxiolytics may be used for achieving symptom control, with side effects monitoring. For cases with severe BPSD, arrangement for inpatient treatment may be necessary. Education and support for the caregivers are made available. The need for rehabilitation is addressed according to the multidisciplinary team's assessment and the setting for such interventions (e.g., daycare center, day hospital) determined on a case-by-case basis. The legal needs of the incapacitated patient on making healthcare choices are addressed through the Guardianship Order framework.

Presently, traditional Chinese medicine (TCM) plays a relatively minor role in dementia treatment in Hong Kong, although clinical trials on the role of herbal agents (e.g., curcumin and others) are underway. The role of "mind–body exercises" [4], a non-pharmacological treatment with reported efficacy in preserving memory in older adults, remains to be explored (see also Chapter 8B on non-pharmacological approaches).

Approach to patients with dementia II: in the China mainland

National level (not applicable to Hong Kong)

A compendium of treatment guidelines for dementia [5] was published by the Ministry of Health of the People's Republic of China, the Chinese Society of Psychiatry, and the Chinese Center for Disease Control and Prevention in July 2006. It emphasizes a comprehensive approach towards patients with dementia, including consideration of differential diagnoses, use of radiological, blood, and other investigations, correct subtyping using the ICD-10 criteria, multidisciplinary assessment on the health care, and residential and legal needs. In the section on potential drug treatments, AChEIs and memantine were listed along with antioxidants, vasodilators, calcium channel blockers, alpha blockers, nicotinamides, inositols, and neuropeptides. Antipsychotics, anxiolytics, and antidepressants were recommended to be used as necessary.

It should be pointed out that at this time the only AChEI subsidized nationally is huperzine A (Hup A) [6], an agent not very commonly used outside China. There are currently no specific guidelines on whether drugs should be given at certain phases of the disease or recommendations on whether drugs should be given in combinations or introduced individually. Memantine has been available to most psychiatric facilities since the end of 2006.

Beijing, Shanghai, and other major coastal cities

Huperzine A is much more often used than other AChEIs like donepezil or rivastigmine in the treatment of dementia. It is an alkaloid isolated from the Chinese herb *huperzia serrata*, and is a reversible inhibitor of acetylcholinesterase. In animal studies it was reported that Hup A may pass through the blood–brain barrier more readily than donepezil and rivastigmine, and may have antioxidant properties [6]. Open studies show its potential efficacy in improving memory deficits in elderly subjects with benign senescent forgetfulness and AD [7]. In the Chinese medical literature, a randomized placebo-control trial on AD in 2002 involving 202 subjects with mild and moderate AD revealed significant improvement on the MMSE and ADAS-Cog over a study period of 12 weeks [8]. The reported side effects were bilateral ankle edema, and insomnia in 3% of the subjects. There have been, however, no head-to-head comparisons with donepezil, rivastigmine, or galatamine in human studies, and data from longer-term studies are needed to clear the current controversies concerning the extent of Hup A's benefits to patients with AD [9].

Though conspicuously absent in the named national treatment guidelines for dementia [5], TCM is commonly used in the treatment of dementia symptoms. In fact, geriatric medicine was little developed until the 1980s [10] and TCM has been the standard medical treatment for many centuries. Moreover, according to the "Ninth Five Year Plan for National Economic and Social Development and the Long-Range Objectives to the Year 2010," one of the primary objectives in healthcare development include "attaching equal importance to traditional Chinese Medicine and Western Medicine" [11].

Reports of successful relief of dementia symptoms by TCM are found in the literature [12–16]. Traditional Chinese medicine conceptualizes dementia as a consequence of problems in the "five organs" (heart, liver, spleen, lung, and kidney); imbalance between the yin and yang results in impaired function in these organs [12]. In addition to herbal agents, acupuncture has been used as a means to restore the imbalance between yin and yang [12,17,18]. Not uncommonly, TCM and Western pharmacotherapies are used in combination for this chronic disorder, with variable degrees of success [19].

Non-urbanized areas

There has been no systematic reporting of the care approach by practitioners (a combination of both TCM practitioners and "bare-foot doctors," i.e., physicians with less intensive medical training) servicing the rural areas, where most of the elderly in China dwell. Elderly in the countryside are generally supported by the family, usually the eldest son. Access to modern medicine is generally limited; combined with the poor financial status of most rural inhabitants, and the common perception that dementia is merely part of "normal aging," the persons with dementia may just be ignored by the relatives, unless BPSD are manifested. For persons with psychotic symptoms, the traditional construct is that they have fallen prey to spirit possession [10], and exorcism and as a consequence psychiatric treatment may not be sought. In addition, the presence of BPSD, which may not be understood as a medical condition, could potentially lead to elder abuse and other forms of maltreatment.

Fortunately, there are clearly outlined governmental plans to improve the health situation in the rural areas (as outlined in Chapter 7C on care arrangements for dementia in China).

Future developments

It is hoped that with the publication of treatment guidelines, dementia treatment may become more standardized. Traditional therapeutic measures should be examined within the modern clinical trial framework. In addition, the impact of policies which attend to the legal and ethical needs of the dementia patient will certainly create a significant public health impact in a nation with a very rapidly aging population.

References

1. World Health Organization. *The ICD-10 Classification of Mental and Behavioural Disorders. Diagnostic Criteria for Research.* Geneva, World Health Organization, 1993.
2. American Psychiatric Association. *Diagnostic and Statistical Manual of Mental Disorders*, 4th edn. Washington, DC, American Psychiatric Association, 1994.
3. Boothby LA, Doering PL. Vitamin C and vitamin E for Alzheimer's disease. *Ann Pharmacother* 2005; **39**(12): 2073–80.
4. Chan AS, Ho Y, Cheung M, *et al.* Association between mind-body and cardiovascular exercises and memory in older adults. *J Am Geriatr Soc* 2005; **53**(10): 1754–60.
5. Ministry of Health. *The Chinese Guidelines for Dementia Therapies*. Beijing, Government of the People's Republic of China, 2006.
6. Zangara A. The psychopharmacology of huperzine A: an alkaloid with cognitive enhancing and neuroprotective properties of interest in the treatment of Alzheimer's disease. *Pharmacol Biochem Behav* 2003; **75**(3): 675–86.
7. Wang R, Yan H, Tang XC. Progress in studies of huperzine A, a natural cholinesterase inhibitor from Chinese herbal medicine. *Acta Pharmacol Sin* 2006; **27**(1): 1–26.
8. Zhang Z, Wang X, Chen Q, *et al.* [Clinical efficacy and safety of huperzine Alpha in the treatment of mild to moderate Alzheimer disease, a placebo-controlled, double-blind, randomized trial.] *Nat Med J China* 2002; **82**(14): 941–4.

9. Lyketsos CG, Colenda CC, Beck C, *et al.* Position statement of the American Association for Geriatric Psychiatry regarding principles of care for patients with dementia resulting from Alzheimer disease. *Am J Geriatr Psychiatry* 2006; **14**(7): 561–72.
10. Ineichen B. Influences on the care of demented elderly people in the People's Republic of China. *Int J Geriatr Psychiatry* 1998; **13**(2): 122–6.
11. Chiu H, Zhang M. Services for dementia in the developing world: A Chinese view. In: O'Brien J, Ames D, Burns A, eds. *Dementia*. London, Arnold. 2000; 344–8.
12. Sun GL, Ren JL, Sun QJ. Progress in clinical study of senile dementia. *J Tradit Chin Med* 1997; **38**: 628–30.
13. Wu L, Cheng SY, Wang Q, Chen YB. [Advances in study on the pharmacological effects of active components of Chinese herbs on Alzheimer's disease.] *Zhongguo Zhong Yao Za Zhi* 2004; **29**(5): 387–9.
14. Sun G, Ren J, Sun Q. Advances in TCM treatment of senile dementia. *J Tradit Chin Med* 1999; **19**(4): 304–12.
15. Oishi M, Mochizuki Y, Takasu T, Chao E, Nakamura S. Effectiveness of traditional Chinese medicine in Alzheimer disease. *Alzheimer Dis Assoc Disord* 1998; **12**(3): 247–50.
16. Wang X, Zhai M. Experience in TCM treatment of senile dementia. *J Tradit Chin Med* 1996; **16**(4): 299–303.
17. Chen ZH, Lai XS, Jiang GH. [Effects of electro-acupuncture on electroencephalography in patients with vascular dementia.] *Zhongguo Zhong Xi Yi Jie He Za Zhi* 2006; **26**(8): 738–40.
18. Yu J, Zhang X, Liu C, Meng Y, Han J. Effect of acupuncture treatment on vascular dementia. *Neurol Res* 2006; **28**(1): 97–103.
19. Guo XZ, Zhang HC, Cao JG, Wang Y, Wang J. Clinical study on treating dementia with combined traditional Chinese medicine and Western medicine. *Shanxi Med J* 2003; **32**(5): 425–7.

Raising global awareness: the role of non-governmental organizations

Alzheimer's Disease International

Marc Wortmann

Introduction

While some individuals and research groups are very familiar with the extraordinary projected growth in the numbers of people with dementia and its social and healthcare implications, they are equally conscious of the lack of knowledge more widely, including amongst key policy makers, and consequently the crucial importance of raising awareness at all levels. Typically this awareness effort has been led by national or more local Alzheimer associations, organizations that have sprung up in many countries around the world over the last two decades. The first Alzheimer association was founded in Canada in 1977, followed closely by the USA, UK, Australia, and Japan. From the beginning of the 1980s we have seen similar organizations being established in (Western) Europe. In 1984 a group of people involved in these national associations came together in Washington DC to start an international umbrella body namely, Alzheimer's Disease International (ADI). By 2010 the number of ADI members had risen to 73, with one member association per country and ADI is now one of the broadest representative international patient and service organizations.

Awareness

A good friend of mine once said that campaigning is like Einstein's $e = mc^2$ where the impact in raising general awareness is a function of funding (or mass m) and creativity (c). As most Alzheimer associations do not have the resources to produce and finance massive million dollar campaigns, they have to be very creative to attract attention and fortunately the latter can be particularly effective in achieving overall impact.

Dementia: A Global Approach, ed. Ennapadam S. Krishnamoorthy, Martin J. Prince, and Jeffrey L. Cummings. Published by Cambridge University Press.

But there is a preliminary issue. When we talk about awareness, what do we mean? Dementia, in many parts of the world, is still a highly stigmatized disease. Even as recently as May 31, 2007 in Houston, James Watson, Nobel Prize winner and discoverer of the DNA structure, was presented with his individual DNA genome. It confirmed an increased risk for cancer, but he declined the opportunity to discover the odds he faces for developing Alzheimer's disease[1].

Raising awareness can be pursued at many different levels: amongst individuals and communities, within professional healthcare circles, amongst governments and policy makers, or amongst society as a whole.

On an individual level it has to do with accepting and gaining insight into the disease. This is an issue for the person with dementia, the caregiver, and the primary physician and this interrelationship differs for each individual. Alzheimer associations do not intervene in this process, but can facilitate it by giving support to caregivers through information on how to cope with the disease, setting up caregiver training, and organizing support groups both for caregivers and people with dementia. There are many formats for these activities, but one creative approach that combines both information and support is the Alzheimer Café, developed in the Netherlands in the late 1990s and now emerging in many other countries. The Café is held monthly in an informal setting and is a forum for discussion. Topics discussed range from how to recognize dementia, the importance of a diagnosis, how to cope with the disease at home, to respite and institutional care and legal issues. The unusual combination of the Café concept with Alzheimer's disease raises awareness of the disease and reduces stigma. This is particularly effective on a local level as this novel scheme provides local groups with the opportunity to attract interest from newspapers and other media.

Raising awareness amongst health professionals – primary care physicians, mental health workers, home care and nursing home staff – presents us with one of our greatest challenges. Having worked in the field of Alzheimer associations for more than seven years now, barely a week has passed without people raising it with me. The difficulty faced by primary care physicians is that they see few people with dementia in their practice every year, and then often only for a brief consultation. Many primary care physicians believe that they have little to offer a patient with dementia as there is no magic pill yet to cure the disease. Furthermore, other healthcare workers often have little knowledge and understanding of the disease. There is, of course, an easy way to solve this problem through the direct education of health professionals. However, as long as education about dementia is not a formal part of the curriculum, we must supplement this program with our own teaching activities. The annual ADI international conference, national conferences, symposia, and training courses that are currently organized by more-established ADI members have proved effective ways to address this problem.

Finally, the challenge of spreading the word about dementia throughout societies as a whole is a very interesting topic, which builds on aspects of raising awareness noted above. One of ADI's greatest achievements has been the foundation and development of

Ich habe
2 Töchter
Handeln, wenn Erinnerungen verblassen.
Denn zunehmende Vergesslichkeit kann ein
Anzeichen für eine Alzheimer-Erkrankung sein.
Wenn Sie Hilfe brauchen, rufen Sie uns an.
Alzheimer-Telefon 0 18 03 / 17 10 17 (9 cent/min)
helfen nicht vergessen
Deutsche Alzheimer Gesellschaft e. V.
www.helfen-nicht-vergessen.de
Schirmherrin: Renate Schmidt, Bundesministerin für Familie, Senioren, Frauen und Jugend

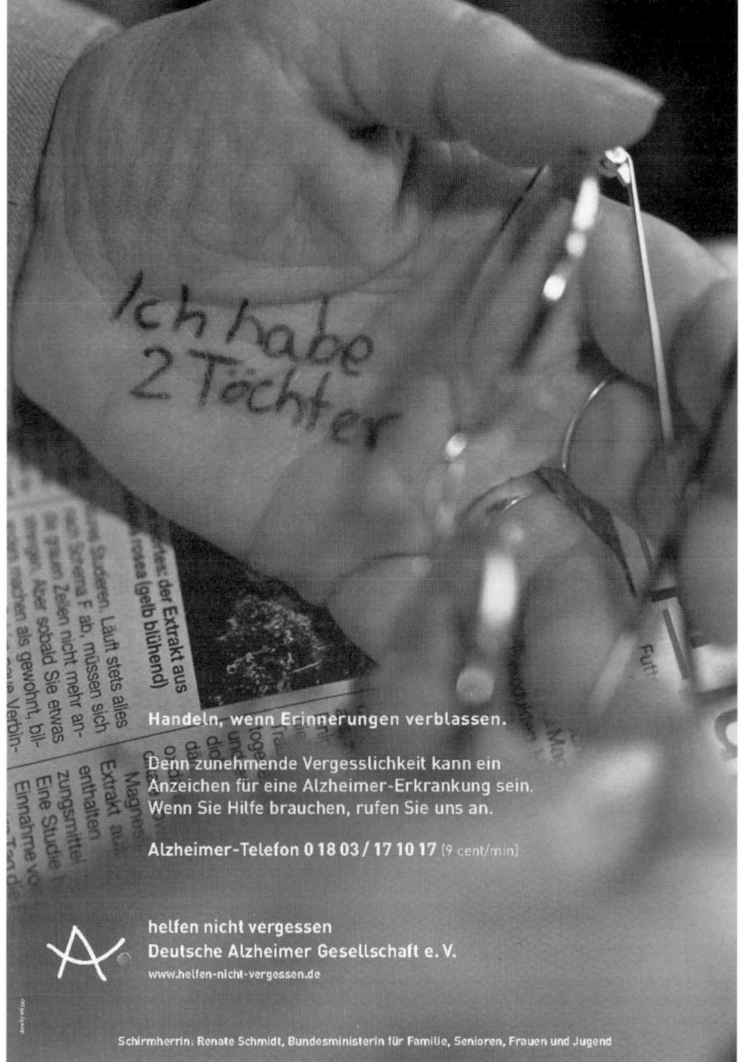

Figure 10A.1 Germany. Reproduced with permission.

World Alzheimer's Day (September 21), a day of international solidarity against dementia which is formally recognized by the World Health Organization. Starting in a small way in 1994, the recognition of this day has grown gradually internationally to the huge participatory event it is today. Each year more than 100 000 caregivers, people with dementia, volunteers, and professionals get involved in all kinds of activities to mark the event. These range from away-days for people with dementia and their families, symposia, music or theater performances (for example in the Theatre La Scala in Milan in Italy every year) to fundraising events and media interviews. However, by far the most popular event

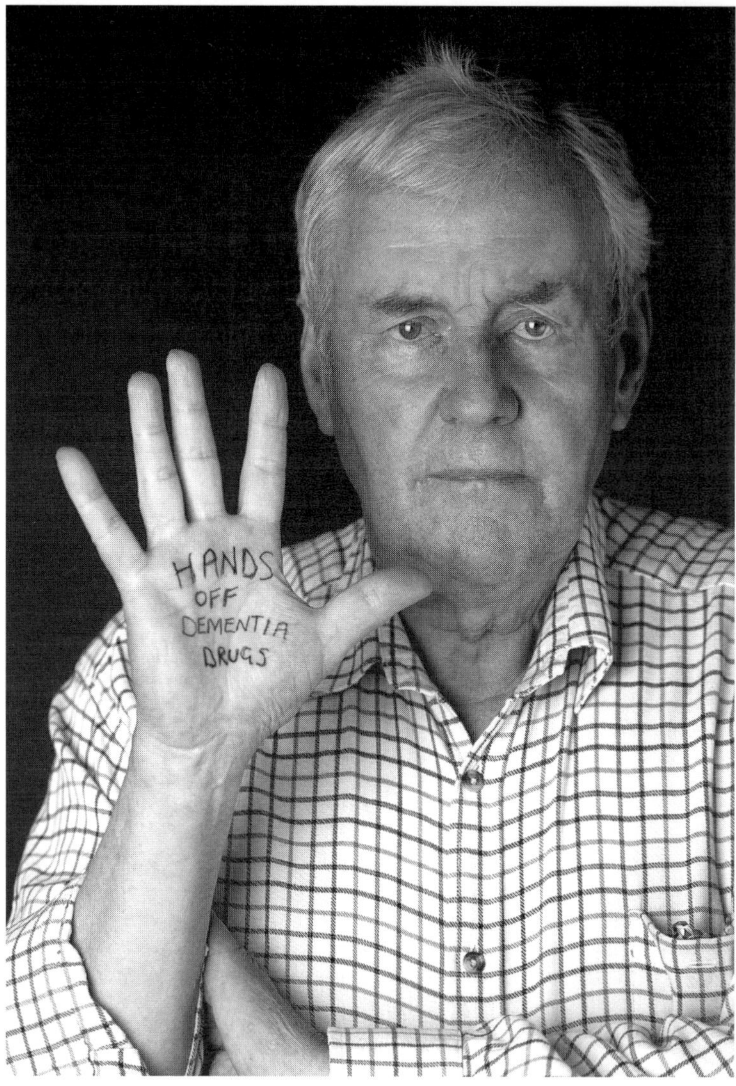

Figure 10A.2 UK. Reproduced with permission.

worldwide to commemorate World Alzheimer's Day is a Memory Walk. This event began in 1989 in the USA, when nine chapters of the Alzheimer Association organized Memory Walks in their own regions. Since then the idea has spread throughout the rest of the USA and worldwide and now more than 500 Memory Walks are held in the USA alone and hundreds more around the rest of the world.

Influencing policy makers

It is not easy to persuade policy makers to place dementia firmly on their agenda. One of the

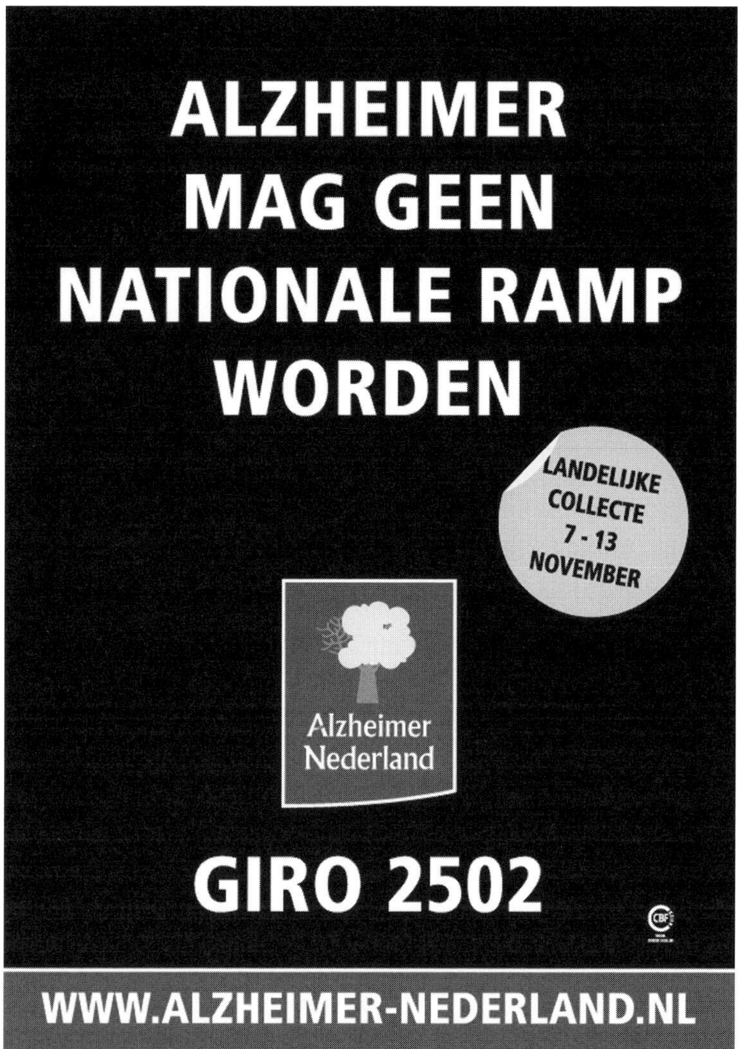

Figure 10A.3 The Netherlands. Reproduced with permission.

founders of ADI, Jerry Stone from Chicago, once told me a story about the start of the American association. He went to Congress to meet some politicians and to ask them to pay attention to dementia. They said to him, "Is this really an issue? Do the papers write about it?" So he went to the journalists and they asked him, "Do they talk about it on Capitol Hill?" It is a vicious circle but one that shows that tackling public awareness at a number of levels is necessary before policy makers react to the issue. In close collaboration with its 10/66

Dementia Research Group, ADI recently decided to approach the World Health Organization to put dementia on its agenda as a global health priority.

Examples of national campaigns

National Alzheimer associations have run a variety of awareness campaigns within their countries, many of which have been extremely successful.

Germany ran a very effective campaign a few years ago: "*Helfen nicht vergessen*" or "don't forget to help." The central image for the campaign was a hand with a written message on it (see Figure 10A.1). These images were used for posters and advertisements, and on the campaign website people were asked to send pictures with text written on their own hands. Over 10 000 people participated in the campaign.

A few years later the Alzheimer Society in the *UK* tried to influence policy makers to reimburse drugs for dementia using the same concept (Figure 10A.2).

In the *Netherlands* an awareness campaign started in 2002. Large posters at train stations and other public places spread the message: "Alzheimer's should not become a national disaster" (Figure 10A.3). Even though some considered the campaign too negative, politicians and policy makers were stimulated to approach the Dutch association to ask how they could contribute.

The association in *Brazil* managed to secure a TV-spot produced and broadcasted for free, thanks to the help of a well-known actress. The 30-second feature was sent to all TV-stations, many of whom showed it, helping to raise awareness.

The Fundación Alzheimer *Venezuela* raised awareness by producing a fashion calendar with information about dementia and the work of the association.

Securing celebrity support is an effective way of raising profile and awareness as it provides an attractive media hook. Finding celebrities to champion the cause can be difficult, however, as dementia is not generally a popular charity.

The Alzheimer's Association in the *USA* recently launched a new campaign to educate and promote a healthy lifestyle: Maintain Your Brain. This is a new approach because it has a much more positive slant and reflects on the individual's own responsibility and capacity to ward off dementia.

Conclusion

Raising awareness about dementia has a long way to go to match the more established health issues in the public mind of cancer, cardiovascular disease, and HIV/AIDS for example. But by applying a range of awareness-raising techniques and linking this to information about preventive opportunities and strategies, I am confident that through the mutually supportive activities of ADI and its member associations we can raise dementia to an equivalent international priority status.

Reference

1. NRC Handelsblad (NL) October 13, 2007, p. 45.

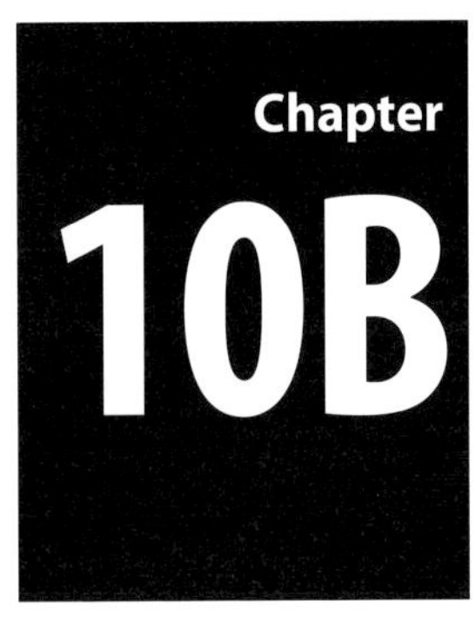

Raising global awareness: the role of non-governmental organizations

Perspectives from a developing nation

Jacob Roy Kuriakose

Introduction

With increasing longevity, the number of people with dementia is increasing exponentially. Of the many diseases that humanity faces today, Alzheimer's disease is perhaps the cruelest and most debilitating. It strips the person of all that they have achieved in their lifetime leaving them a pale shadow of their original selves. Those affected are often helpless, dependent totally on their caregivers. With globalization and rapid urbanization, care of the elderly, particularly those with dementia, poses a major burden in most societies. While there is need for better awareness which could help in early identification and developing coping strategies, the situation is rather grim in most developing countries. This is mainly due to ignorance, lack of resources, trained man power, and facilities.

The great strength in most developing countries is the family support, which over the years has been threatened by urbanization and migration of younger people looking for better opportunities. Women who used to be traditional caregivers for elders in the family have started taking up jobs outside their homes; leaving a vacuum. Finding a viable alternative source to take up this responsibility is difficult.

Alzheimer's disease, a most dreaded illness of old age, now rivals other major diseases like cancer and HIV/AIDS in evoking fright and helplessness among patients and their families. Yet, there is lack of awareness among the general population regarding the existence of this devastating illness, which often transcends to include health professionals. It is believed that thousands of patients with Alzheimer's disease remain undetected and undiagnosed. Creating mass awareness, sensitizing and training the medical and health personnel is the top priority in meeting the challenge of Alzheimer's disease.

Awareness in the community

Broadly we should address this for three core sections in a community, i.e., family, friends,

Dementia: A Global Approach, ed. Ennapadam S. Krishnamoorthy, Martin J. Prince, and Jeffrey L. Cummings. Published by Cambridge University Press.

and neighbors. Family support is primary in providing quality care to a person with dementia. Apart from the primary caregivers other family members also need to know what Alzheimer's disease is and what it implies to the person and his/ her family.

Family members need to be made aware of the symptoms of Alzheimer's disease and the need for them to provide both practical and emotional support to the caregiver. It is important for them to accept the person with Alzheimer's disease, the way he/she is and not the way they want him/her to be. If the caregiver is educated on various aspects of the disease, then he/she in turn can disseminate that knowledge within the family. The family should be open to suggestions and may seek the help of the local chapter of the Alzheimer's Society for more information and support.

Knowledgeable friends too can play an important role. The caregiver may ventilate frustrations and problems with them. A friend knowledgeable about dementia can be an emotional safety belt. Neighbors once they become knowledgeable about dementia can provide a lot of support. Even enquiring about the patient and wellness of the caregiver has a significant impact. They can also help the families at times of hospitalization or during emergency. A knowledgeable sympathetic neighbor can be a crucial source of help during any crisis.

Role of non-governmental organizations

Non-governmental organizations (NGOs) can play a great role in disseminating information and create better awareness about dementia. The NGO directly charged with this role and responsibility is the National Alzheimer's Society, which should play a lead role. Other NGOs that play an important role include organizations dedicated to care of the elderly; service organizations like Rotary, Lions, etc.; senior citizens forums; philanthropic trusts and foundations. All such organizations can take an active part in such dementia awareness programs at local, regional, national, and international levels. They could undertake a number of programs such as:

- Organizing talks and seminars
- Publication of information in simple language
- Liasion with hospitals and other health-related organizations
- Develop a network
- Address corporate houses for funding
- Effective media relations.

Success of a program initiated by a NGO largely depends on the passion and commitment with which they address the problems of dementia. Involving knowledgeable caregivers shall be an added advantage. Enlisting the support of volunteers is important. It is important to ensure that adequate training is imparted to these volunteers and that their roles are clearly defined.

Awareness programs should start at all levels, from schools to universities, large companies, service organizations, hospitals and other health institutions, and media houses. In schools information about dementia could be given in simple language, whereas in colleges details of caregiving could be given. Staff of old age homes should be trained to look for warning signs of dementia among the residents.

Alzheimer's Disease International (ADI) is the world Federation of nearly 75 national dementia organizations. Raising awareness of dementia globally is one of its main activities. September 21 is being observed as *World Alzheimer's Day*. This has helped in focusing worldwide attention on the growing problem of dementia. The national chapters of ADI (Alzheimer's and Related Disorders Society of India for example) can develop hub–spoke relationships with a wide range of NGOs working with dementia sufferers. By providing these NGOs with training and access to high-quality educational material it will be possible to disseminate quality information to a wide audience.

Disseminating information can be most effectively done by doctors and other health professionals. They could demystify dementia, bringing about greater acceptance among the community about the status of dementia as an organic illness on par with cancer, stroke, heart disease, and other major killer diseases. There are several myths about dementia. Both print and electronic media can bring out real-life stories and how families struggle to cope and manage the situation. Networking with hospitals and professional organizations of doctors will help Alzheimer's societies to develop skills in creating better awareness. Training of primary care physicians in early diagnosis, and details of the currently available interventions (pharmacological and non-pharmacological) is important. By sponsoring seminars or workshops on the recent advances in dementia care and research, as part of their national conferences, Alzheimer's disease societies can create better awareness and visibility of the cause. Disseminating accurate information on the available services in the country like memory clinics, daycare centers, home care programs, respite care and helplines is also very important.

There is a gross shortage of trained manpower in caring for people with dementia all over the world. Organizing such training programs and providing this information will be of great help to the affected families. Training of caregivers, and volunteers helps to add quality to dementia care, which in turn will help in raising awareness. Training programs will include:

- Caregiving tips
- Communication with those affected
- Do's and don'ts in caregiving
- Training in palliative care

Working with government

Efforts are underway to make dementia a health priority in many countries across the world. In order to educate parliamentarians, policy makers and bureaucrats, series of personal meetings, seminars and workshops are of crucial importance. Non-governmental agencies, particularly the National Alzheimer Society, should take the initiative to motivate their respective governments to accept dementia as an important public health problem. There is felt need to make dementia a national health priority and apprise Governments world over about the perceived looming threat of a dementia epidemic that is causing great concern. The success of any national dementia care program will only come through governmental involvement. Only when dementia care becomes an integral part of primary healthcare systems will the benefits reach the common man. The ability to convince Governments and other funding agencies will also depend on our ability to provide facts and figures relevant to that setting, necessitating more local research. Indeed data from local research will enhance the acceptance of the Alzheimer's movement not only with government but also with the medical community, funding agencies and corporate houses.

Conclusion

Alzheimer's disease is as of now incurable. Care of those affected rests to a large extent in the hands of few caregivers, who often suffer in silence leading miserable and stress-filled lives. They often are unaware as to where they should turn for help. Spreading awareness about dementia is like teaching a poor person without any employment skills to fish. Once equipped he/she becomes capable of taking care of his/her needs and that of the affected person, for the sole reason that he/she is now equipped with knowledge that he/she did not previously possess. National Alzheimer's Associations have the potential to empower and emancipate through awareness building and education of people with dementia and their families and are best suited to take up this noble mission at the global level.

Chapter 11

The contribution of cross-cultural research to dementia care and policy: an overview, focusing on the work of the 10/66 Dementia Research Group

Martin J. Prince

Introduction

The 10/66 Dementia Research Group (10/66) was founded in 1998, at the annual conference of Alzheimer's Disease International (ADI), in Cochin, India. 10/66 refers to the less than one-tenth of all population-based research into dementia that had been directed towards the two-thirds or more of people with dementia living in low and middle income countries (LAMIC). The 10/66 Dementia Research Group was formed to redress this imbalance, encouraging active research collaboration between centers in different LAMIC and between developed countries and LAMIC. The Cochin symposium established priorities for the 10/66 Dementia Research Group, described in a consensus publication co-authored by the founding members [1]. More research was needed to describe prevalence and incidence, and to explore regional variations using harmonized methods. Another priority was the description of care arrangements for people with dementia, quantifying the impact upon caregivers of providing care, and evaluating the effectiveness of new services for people with dementia and their caregivers. The group identified potential through good-quality research for generating awareness, pioneering service development, and influencing policy. Now is an opportune time to review progress. This chapter will focus, but not exclusively, upon the work of the 10/66 Dementia Research Group.

The validity of dementia diagnosis across cultures

The validity of methods used in cross-cultural research is fundamental to the success of the enterprise. Without this, informative cross-cultural

Dementia: A Global Approach, ed. Ennapadam S. Krishnamoorthy, Martin J. Prince, and Jeffrey L. Cummings. Published by Cambridge University Press.

comparisons are impossible. Many potential obstacles need to be overcome [2]. Those with little or no education may appear to "fail" on cognitive screening tests even in the absence of cognitive impairment or decline. The task may be unfamiliar to them, or the information requested irrelevant. Tasks involving literacy, numeracy, or drawing are particularly problematic, but in practice any cognitive item for which the probability of a correct response is strongly influenced by education will tend to be biased. Culture, including language, may also influence the salience and feasibility of cognitive items, and their relative difficulty. Cultural influences, as we shall see, may also impact on the assessment of social or occupational disability, since the normal roles of older people may vary considerably between cultures.

The development and validation of the 10/66 dementia diagnosis

Accordingly, between 2000 and 2002, the 10/66 Dementia Research Group carried out pilot studies in 26 centers from 16 LAMIC in Latin America and the Caribbean, Africa, India, Russia, China, and SE Asia. Two thousand eight hundred and eighty-five persons aged 60 and over were interviewed, 729 people with dementia, and three groups free of dementia; 702 with depression, 694 with high education, and 760 with low education [3]. The pilot studies demonstrated the feasibility and validity of a one-phase culture and education-fair diagnostic protocol for population-based research [3,4]. The Geriatric Mental State (a structured clinical interview assessing dementia, depression and psychosis syndromes) [5], the Community Screening Instrument for Dementia (a cognitive test, and informant interview for evidence of intellectual and functional decline) [6], and the modified Consortium to Establish a Registry for Alzheimer's Disease (CERAD) 10-word list-learning task each independently predicted dementia diagnosis [7]. A probabilistic algorithm derived in one-half of the sample from all four of these elements performed better than any of them individually; applied to the other half of the sample it identified 94% of dementia cases with false positive rates of 15%, 3%, and 6% in the depression, high education, and low education groups [3]. This algorithm (the 10/66 dementia diagnosis) was "education-fair" in that the false positive rate among those with low levels of education was low, and "culture-fair" in that equivalent validity was established for a wide variety of countries, languages, and cultures. It therefore provides a sound basis for dementia diagnosis in clinical and population-based research, supported by translations of its constituent measures into many languages (Hindi, Tamil, Malayalam, Konkani, Mandarin/Cantonese, Russian, Spanish, Portuguese) covering the majority of the peoples of the non-English speaking world.

The validity of 10/66 dementia compared with that of DSM-IV dementia

For the 10/66 population-based surveys we decided also to apply the Diagnostic and Statistical Manual of Mental Disorders, Fourth edition (DSM-IV) [8] criteria for dementia, since these were hitherto the most widely applied criteria in studies worldwide. We extended the scope of the one-phase assessment to ensure that the necessary data were recorded, and devised and validated a computerized application of the DSM-IV criteria [9]. Use of these criteria has been associated with strikingly low prevalences of dementia in some previous LAMIC studies [10,11]. Therefore the relative concurrent and predictive validity of the two diagnostic approaches, 10/66 dementia and DSM-IV dementia, needed to be evaluated. Our confidence in the validity of the 10/66 dementia diagnosis was bolstered by the subsequent demonstration, in the course of our population-based study in Cuba, that it agreed better with Cuban clinician diagnoses than did the DSM-IV computerized algorithm, which missed many recent onset and mild cases [9]. However, an essential feature of the dementia syndrome is that it is a progressive neurodegenerative disorder. The principal clinical rationale for an early diagnosis is that it alerts the person concerned and their family to the probability of future deterioration. We therefore assessed the predictive validity of the 10/66 dementia diagnosis in our population-based study sample in Chennai, South India, in a three-year follow-up of all those with DSM-IV dementia, 10/66 dementia, mild cognitive impairment (MCI), and "cognitive impairment no dementia" (CIND) at baseline [12]. The hypothesis for predictive validity was that true cases would have progressed, in cognitive impairment, functional disability, and needs for care. We traced 54 of those with 10/66 dementia at baseline of whom 25 (46.3%) had died, double the mortality rate among those with MCI and CIND. Twenty-two of the 24 people with 10/66 dementia that were reexamined still met 10/66 dementia criteria. There was clear evidence of clinical progression and increased needs for care. Only one "case" had unambiguously improved. Cognitive function had deteriorated and disability increased to a much greater extent than among those with MCI or CIND. The strong predictive validity of the 10/66 dementia diagnosis was consistent with a lack of sensitivity of the DSM-IV criteria to mild to moderate cases, and, thus, with the notion that it may underestimate prevalence in less developed regions.

The prevalence of dementia

The *Lancet*/ADI estimates of the global prevalence of dementia

In 2004, ADI convened a panel of international experts to review the global evidence on the prevalence of dementia, and to estimate the prevalence of dementia in each world region, the current numbers of people affected, and the projected increases over time. The results were published in the *Lancet* in 2005. In 2001, 24.2 million people lived with dementia worldwide, with 4.6 million new cases annually [13] (similar to the global incidence of non-fatal stroke [14]). Two-thirds of all people with dementia lived in LAMIC. Numbers were predicted to double every 20 years to over 80 million by 2040, with much sharper increases in low and middle income compared with high income countries. These projected increases were accounted for solely by the different patterns of demographic aging (the increase in the absolute and relative numbers of older people), since the age-specific prevalence of dementia was assumed to remain constant over time. A tendency previously noted for prevalence to be somewhat lower in LAMIC than in the developed north [2,10,11] was supported by the consensus judgment of the ADI expert panel, reviewing all evidence available at that time [13]. Differences in survival could only be part of the explanation, as estimates of incidence in some studies [15,16] were also much lower than those reported in the West. However, the *Lancet*/ADI estimates were described as "provisional," given that prevalence data were lacking in many world regions, and patchy in others, with few studies and widely varying estimates [13]. Coverage was good in Europe, North America, and in developed Asia Pacific countries; South Korea, Japan, Taiwan, and Australia. Several studies have been published from India and China, but estimates were too few and/or too variable to provide a consistent overview for these huge countries. There was a particular dearth of published epidemiological studies in Latin America [17–19], Africa [10], Russia, the Middle East, and Indonesia. Therefore, there was a strong reliance upon the consensus judgment of the international panel of experts.

The 10/66 Dementia Research Group prevalence studies

The 10/66 Dementia Research Group subsequently completed population-based surveys (2003–7) of dementia prevalence and impact in 12 sites in 8 LAMIC (India, China, Cuba, Dominican Republic, Brazil, Venezuela, Mexico, and Peru) [20–25], with a second wave of surveys underway in Puerto Rico, Sri Lanka, and South Africa. Cross-sectional comprehensive one-phase surveys were conducted of all residents aged 65 and over of geographically defined catchment areas in each site with a sample size of 2000–3000 in each country. The net result is a unique resource of directly comparable data on over 20 000 older adults from three continents. All studies used the same cross-culturally validated assessments (dementia diagnosis and subtypes, other mental and physical health, anthropometry, demographics, extensive non-communicable disease risk factor questionnaires, disability/functioning, health service utilization, care arrangements, and caregiver strain). A publicly accessible data archive has been established as a resource for the academic community (www.alz.co.uk/1066).

The prevalence of DSM-IV dementia varied widely, from less than 1% in the least developed sites (India and rural Peru) to 6.4% in Cuba [21]. Prevalence of 10/66 dementia was higher than that of DSM-IV dementia, and more consistent across sites, varying between 5.6% and 11.7% [21]. The discrepancy was explained by the observation that informants in the least developed sites, particularly India, were less likely to report cognitive decline and social impairment (an essential criterion for DSM-IV dementia diagnosis) even in the presence of objective memory impairment [21]. Levels of disability as measured by the structured WHODAS 2.0 disability scale were similar for 10/66 dementia cases regardless of whether they were confirmed as cases by the DSM-IV dementia algorithm [21]. After standardizing for age and sex, DSM-IV prevalence was similar in the urban Latin American sites to that in Europe, but in China the prevalence was only one-half, and in India and rural Latin America one-quarter or less of the European prevalence. We concluded that the DSM-IV dementia criteria may have underestimated dementia prevalence, particularly in regions with low awareness of this emerging public health problem.

There are several possible explanations for the discrepancy between objective cognitive impairment and informant reports [21]. First, our cognitive tests may be biased, overestimating cognitive impairment in these settings, but this seems unlikely given the strong evidence of criteria and predictive validity (see above). Second, objective cognitive impairment may be less likely to lead to noticeable impairment in the performance of normal social roles, because of the high levels of instrumental support routinely provided to all older people, particularly in the early stages of dementia. More attention may need to be given to developing culturally relevant assessments to detect the consequences of early intellectual decline. Third, impairment/decline may have been noted by informants, but they may have been reluctant to disclose this because of the culture of respect towards older people (supported by our finding of lower informant report scores for heads of household and male participants [21]). Fourth, low awareness; impairment/decline may have been noted, but attributed to "normal aging" [26,27] and hence not worthy of mention given the implicit focus of the assessments upon abnormality.

The World Alzheimer Report: new estimates of global prevalence of dementia

Since the *Lancet*/ADI estimates were published, the global evidence-base has expanded considerably. There have been new studies from Spain [28,29], Italy [30], and the USA [31]. The exciting development, however, has been an explosion of studies from LAMIC, and other regions and groups previously under-represented in the literature. These included ADI's 10/66 Dementia Research Group studies in Brazil, Cuba, Dominican Republic, Peru, Mexico, Venezuela, India, and China [21,22], and further new prevalence studies from Brazil [32], Peru [33], Cuba [34], Venezuela [35], China [36], Korea [37], India [38], Thailand [39], Australia (indigenous people [40]), Guam [41], Poland [42] and Turkey [43]. The leaders of the *Lancet*/ADI review, Martin Prince and Cleusa Ferri were commissioned in 2008 to assist the World Health Organization (WHO) in updating the global burden of disease (GBD) estimates, by conducting fully systematic reviews of the prevalence and incidence of dementia, and associated mortality, in 21 GBD world regions. This provided an ideal opportunity to revisit the literature, and to assess the extent to which it was possible, in some or all regions, to summarize the evidence on the prevalence of dementia by carrying out quantitative meta-analyses of the available data, rather than relying on expert consensus. Findings from this exercise were published in ADI's 2009 World Alzheimer Report [44].

The systematic review identified 147 prevalence studies worldwide since 1980. A recent marked increase in the number of studies from LAMIC was accompanied by a sharp decline in research in high income countries (Figure 11.1). In many of these countries, the evidence-base is fast becoming out of date.

The quality of many of the included studies was relatively poor. However, there was no difference in the overall quality scores between LAMIC and high income countries, and more recent studies were of higher methodological quality. A particular concern was the 49% of all studies that used, but misapplied a research design with two or more phases. This error is likely to lead to an underestimate of true prevalence [45]. However, for two-phase studies in general, a higher prevalence was observed, probably because of loss to follow-up in the interval between the screening and definitive diagnostic assessments. Furthermore, 57% of all studies

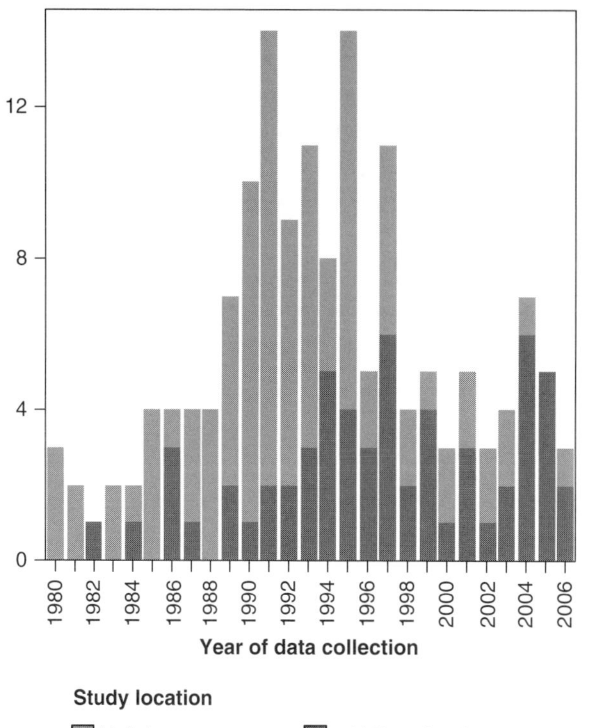

Figure 11.1 Numbers of prevalence studies, by year of data collection and income level of the country where the research was carried out.

lacked a properly comprehensive dementia diagnostic workup.

When compared with our earlier *Lancet*/ADI consensus, after age standardization to the western European population structure, the new estimates of dementia prevalence for all those aged 60 years and over were higher for three regions – Western Europe (7.29% vs. 5.92%), South Asia (5.65% vs. 3.40%), and Latin America (8.50% vs. 7.25%). Those for East Asia were lower (4.98% vs. 6.46%). However, in comparison with the much greater heterogeneity seen in the *Lancet*/ ADI estimates, regional estimates had generally converged (Figure 11.2). While there was a fourfold variation in prevalence overall, from 2.07% (sub-Saharan Africa, West) to 8.50% (Latin America), most of the standardized prevalences lay in a band between 5% and 7%. The major source of variation was clearly the very low estimated prevalence for the four sub-Saharan African regions.

When regional prevalence estimates were applied to population estimates, it was calculated that there were 35.6 million people with dementia worldwide in 2010, the numbers nearly doubling every 20 years, to 65.7 million in 2030 and 115.4 million in 2050. These figures for global prevalence were approximately 10% higher than the earlier *Lancet*/ADI estimates. In 2010, 58% of all people with dementia worldwide lived in LAMIC, rising to 71% by 2050 (Figure 11.3).

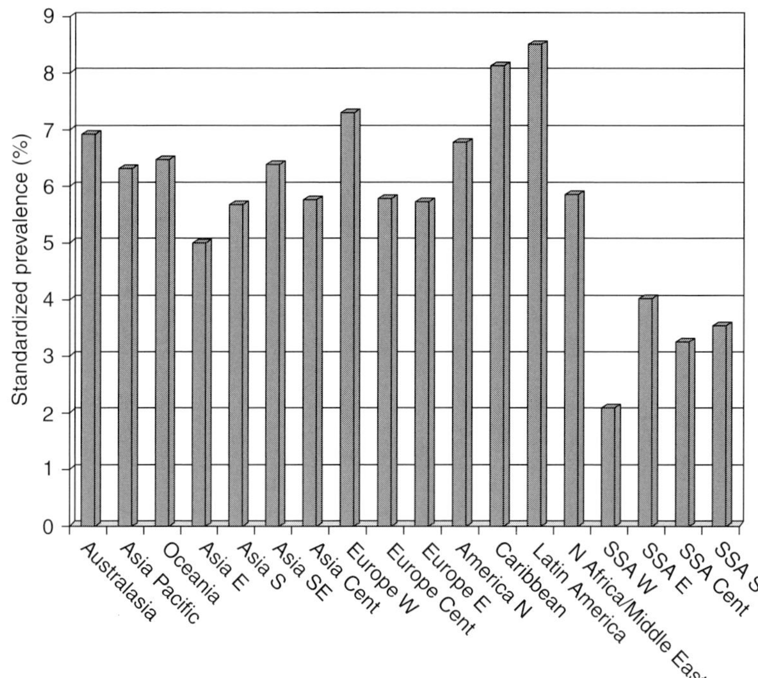

Figure 11.2 Estimated prevalence of dementia (%) for those aged 60 and over, standardized to the western Europe population, by global burden of disease region. SSA, sub-Saharan Africa.

Proportionate increases over the next 20 years in the number of people with dementia will be much steeper in low and middle compared with high income countries. The World Alzheimer Report forecast a 40% increase in numbers in Europe, 63% in North America, 77% in the southern Latin American cone, and 89% in the developed Asia Pacific countries. These figures are to be compared with 117% growth in East Asia, 108% in South Asia, 134–46% in the rest of Latin America, and 125% in North Africa and the Middle East (Table 11.1).

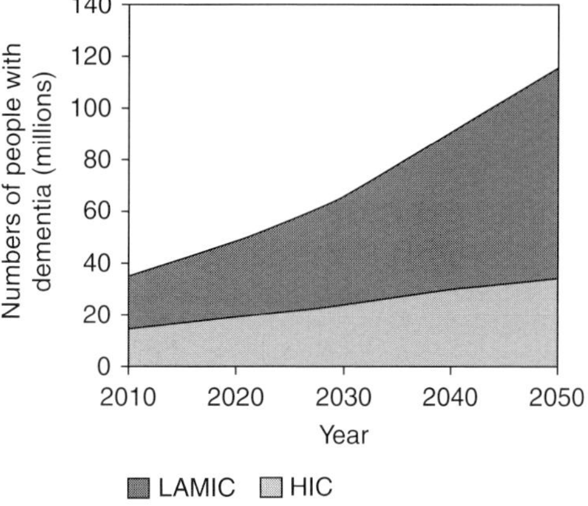

Figure 11.3 The growth in numbers of people with dementia in high income (HIC) and low and middle income countries (LAMIC).

The impact of dementia

Worldwide, surprisingly few epidemiological studies of dementia have gone beyond reporting on prevalence, incidence, and etiology of dementia. The impact of dementia upon the individual, the family, and society has been little studied, particularly its contribution to disability, dependency, caregiver strain, and

Table 11.1 Total population over 60, crude estimated prevalence of dementia (2010), estimated number of people with dementia (2010, 2030, and 2050) and proportionate increases (2010–30 and 2010–50) by global burden of disease world region

GBD region	Over 60 population (millions, 2010)	Crude estimated prevalence (%, 2010)	Number of people with dementia (millions)			Proportionate increases (%)	
			2010	2030	2050	2010–30	2010–50
ASIA	406.55	3.9	15.94	33.04	60.92	107	282
Australasia	4.82	6.4	0.31	0.53	0.79	71	157
Asia Pacific	46.63	6.1	2.83	5.36	7.03	89	148
Oceania	0.49	4.0	0.02	0.04	0.10	100	400
Asia, Central	7.16	4.6	0.33	0.56	1.19	70	261
Asia, East	171.61	3.2	5.49	11.93	22.54	117	311
Asia, South	124.61	3.6	4.48	9.31	18.12	108	304
Asia, Southeast	51.22	4.8	2.48	5.30	11.13	114	349
EUROPE	160.18	6.2	9.95	13.95	18.65	40	87
Europe, Western	97.27	7.2	6.98	10.03	13.44	44	93
Europe, Central	23.61	4.7	1.10	1.57	2.10	43	91
Europe, East	39.30	4.8	1.87	2.36	3.10	26	66
THE AMERICAS	120.74	6.5	7.82	14.78	27.08	89	246
North America	63.67	6.9	4.38	7.13	11.01	63	151

Caribbean	5.06	6.5	0.33	0.62	1.04	88	215
LA, Andean	4.51	5.6	0.25	0.59	1.29	136	416
LA, Central	19.54	6.1	1.19	2.79	6.37	134	435
LA, Southern	8.74	7.0	0.61	1.08	1.83	77	200
LA, Tropical	19.23	5.5	1.05	2.58	5.54	146	428
AFRICA	71.07	2.6	1.86	3.92	8.74	111	370
North Africa/Middle East	31.11	3.7	1.15	2.59	6.19	125	438
SSA, Central	3.93	1.8	0.07	0.12	0.24	71	243
SSA, East	16.03	2.3	0.36	0.69	1.38	92	283
SSA, Southern	4.66	2.1	0.10	0.17	0.20	70	100
SSA, West	15.33	1.2	0.18	0.35	0.72	94	300
WORLD	758.54	4.7	35.56	65.69	115.38	85	225

From *The World Alzheimer Report 2009* [44], with permission.

costs. The response of health services and systems has also been relatively neglected.

Care arrangements and carer strain

In the 10/66 Dementia Research Group pilot study in 26 centers in Latin America, China, India, and Nigeria, we interviewed 706 persons with dementia, and their caregivers [46–48]. Most caregivers were women, living with the person with dementia in extended family households. One-quarter to one-half of households included a child. Larger households were associated with lower carer strain, where the carer was coresident. However, despite the traditional apparatus of family care, levels of carer strain were at least as high as in the developed world. Many had cut back on work to care and faced the additional expense of paid carers and health services. Families from the poorest countries were particularly likely to have used expensive private medical services, and to be spending more than 10% of the per capita Gross National Product on health care. We concluded that the high levels of family strain identified in this study feed into the cycle of disadvantage and should thus be a concern for policy makers in the developing world.

All over the world, the family remains the cornerstone of care for older people who have lost the capacity for independent living. In developed countries with their comprehensive health- and social care systems the vital caring role of families, and their need for support, is often overlooked. In LAMIC the reliability and universality of the family care system is often overestimated [49,50]. A preliminary comparative analysis of the circumstances of those with dementia in each 10/66 Dementia Research Group population-based study site (Table 11.2) highlighted some of the vulnerabilities of dependent older people living in these regions [51]. Social protection is hard to define, depending on an interaction between health status and dependency on the one hand, income sufficiency and secure living arrangements on the other. In the Dominican Republic, rural Peru and Mexico, rural China and in India, pension coverage is low and many people with dementia are significantly reliant on family cash transfers. In contrast with developed countries, it is relatively unusual for people with dementia to live alone or just with their spouse; living with children or children-in-law is the norm, and three-generation households (including children under 16) are relatively common. Nevertheless, around one-fifth of people with dementia (10% to 37% by center) were classified as having potentially vulnerable living circumstances. Many need long-term care, currently provided by family carers. Primary care services do not meet their needs. Governments neither provide long-term care nor support carers.

Behavioral and psychological symptoms of dementia (BPSD)

In the 10/66 Dementia Research Group pilot study, at least one behavioral symptom of dementia (BSD) was reported in 70.9% and at least one psychiatric syndrome was exhibited by 49.5% of the 555 people with dementia included in this substudy [52]. Depression syndromes (43.8%) were most common, followed by anxiety neurosis (14.2%) and schizophreniform/paranoid psychosis (10.9%). More advanced dementia, poorer functioning, and the presence of depression or anxiety were each associated

Table 11.2 Social protection for older people with dementia – 10/66 catchment area surveys in Latin America, India, and China

		Income security				**Secure living arrangements**			**Availability of family support**		
Population-based center catchment area	n	Government or occupational pension	Income from family transfers	Disability pension	Food insecurity	Living alone	Living with spouse only	Total	No children	No children within 50 miles	Total
Cuba (urban)	323	81.4%	7.4%	0.9%	5.6%	6.3%	10.2%	16.5%	16.5%	3.0%	19.5%
Dominican Republic (urban)	242	27.3%	23.6%	0.8%	13.7%	8.5%	10.2%	18.7%	12.0%	13.1%	25.1%
Venezuela (urban)	146	41.1%	2.7%	4.1%	2.7%	5.7%	4.9%	10.6%	7.8%	5.6%	13.4%
Peru (Urban)	130	58.5%	5.4%	1.1%	1.6%	1.6%	9.4%	11.0%	16.4%	0.0%	16.4%
Peru (Rural)	36	66.7%	0.0%	0.0%	8.6%	13.9%	8.3%	22.2%	19.4%	5.7%	25.1%
Mexico (Urban)	93	78.5%	7.5%	1.1%	3.2%	14.0%	9.3%	23.3%	4.3%	0.0%	4.3%
Mexico (Rural)	87	34.5%	17.2%	2.3%	12.6%	16.5%	11.1%	27.6%	4.6%	1.2%	5.8%
China (Urban)	84	84.5%	11.9%	0.0%	0.0%	2.5%	34.5%	37.0%	0.0%	0.0%	0.0%
China (Rural)	56	10.7%	23.2%	0.0%	3.6%	3.6%	8.9%	12.5%	3.6%	4.2%	7.8%
India (Urban)	75	13.3%	28.0%	2.7%	28.0%	4.0%	13.3%	17.3%	5.3%	0.0%	15.3%
India (Rural)	108	26.9%	44.4%	0.0%	17.6%	15.1%	5.7%	20.8%	8.3%	2.6%	10.9%

Modified from Prince [51].

with BSD. Behavioral Symptoms of dementia, and psychiatric syndromes (anxiety neurosis and schizophreniform/paranoid psychosis) independently predicted carer strain after controlling for cognitive impairment. Behavioral and psychological symptoms of dementia are poorly understood, leading to shame and blame. They may be taken by outsiders as prima facie evidence of neglect or abuse. Carers then face a double jeopardy: the strain of care heightened by the stigma and blame that are attached to them because of the disturbed behavior of their relative. It seems that BPSD are common among people with dementia in LAMIC. Representative population studies are needed to clarify prevalence and impact, but our research suggested considerable unmet need, with much scope for intervention.

The impact of dementia relative to that of other chronic diseases

In addition to dementia, the 10/66 one-phase surveys include ascertainment of depression, other mental disorders, hypertension, dyslipidemia, diabetes, metabolic syndrome, heart disease, stroke, chronic obstructive pulmonary disease, and arthritis [20]. As well as providing a rich baseline for studying the etiology of dementia in the incidence phase, this allows exploration of the relative, independent, and interactive contributions of these various chronic conditions to disability, dependency, carer strain, service utilization, economic costs, and mortality. The findings from the first of these analyses, on the independent contributions of chronic diseases to disability [53] were contrary to the GBD report, which cites blindness and deafness as the two leading contributors to years lived with disability among older people in LAMIC. In our analysis, other than in rural India, dementia made the largest contribution to disability, with a median population attributable fraction of 25.5% (range across sites 19.3% to 43.5%). Other substantial contributors were limb impairment (11.7%, 5.6%–34.0%), stroke (11.5%, 2%–21.2%), arthritis (9.9%, 2.8%–35.0%), depression (8.3%, 0.5%–22.9%), eyesight (5.7%, 0%–17.6%), and gastrointestinal impairments (5.1%, 0%–23.2%). These findings suggest that chronic diseases of the brain and mind deserve greater prioritization. Aside from disability, they lead to dependency and present stressful, complex long-term challenges to carers. Societal costs are enormous [54]. Evidence from population-based research on aging and dementia from LAMIC should help to stimulate a wider debate about older people's health and social care needs, and how they should be met [50].

Awareness of dementia in LAMIC

Knowledge, attitudes, and beliefs regarding dementia are best assessed through qualitative research studies. Three studies from India [26,27,55] (two conducted by the 10/66 Dementia Research Group) used a mixture of focus group discussion and open-ended interviews to investigate these issues. They tended to agree regarding the extent of awareness in the different communities studied. First, the typical features of dementia are widely recognized, and indeed named "Chinnan" (literally childishness) in Malayalam language in Kerala [26], "nerva frakese" (tired brain) in Konkani language in Goa [27], and "weak brain" in Hindi in

Banares [55].However, in none of these settings was there any awareness of dementia as an organic brain syndrome, or indeed as any kind of medical condition. Rather, it was perceived as a normal, anticipated part of aging. In Goa, the likely causes were cited as "neglect by family members, abuse, tension and lack of love" [27]. In Kerala, it was reported that most caregivers tended to misinterpret symptoms of the disease and to designate these as deliberate misbehavior by the person with dementia [26]. This general lack of awareness has important consequences. First, there is no structured training on the recognition and management of dementia at any level of the health service. Second, in the absence of understanding regarding its origins, dementia is stigmatized: for example, sufferers are specifically excluded from residential care, and often denied admission to hospital facilities [27]. Third, there is no constituency to place pressure on the government or policy makers to start to provide more responsive dementia care services [26]. Fourth, while families are the main carers, they must do so with little or no support or understanding from other individuals or agencies. A critical mass of informed carers can assist awareness-raising, provide advice and support to families, and can work with Alzheimer associations to lobby for more services that better meet their needs. Community solidarity can effect change through support for policies based on equity and justice – a fairer distribution of healthcare services, and access to effective care regardless of age. Aware communities can provide support, or at least not stigmatize and exclude those with dementia and those who care for them.

Service development and evaluation

People with dementia and their families are particularly unlikely to access health care, despite the high levels of associated disability and carer strain [56]. However, lack of help-seeking should not be presumed to reflect a lack of need. Shaji *et al.*, working with the 10/66 Dementia Research Group in Kerala, Southern India carried out qualitative research with carers of the 17 older persons with Alzheimer's disease:

> Many caregivers expressed a wish to know more about the disease and its management. Most said that they would be interested to attend meetings of support groups or training programs for caregivers. However, none of the people with dementia were in regular contact with any health care facility. Visits to outpatient care facilities were perceived as neither feasible nor useful. None of the caregivers ever received any advice from anybody regarding management of their relatives at home. They said that they were learning from their own experience and were unhappy not to be receiving any help from health professionals. [26].

In Goa too, primary healthcare doctors said that they were not consulted, and had little or no direct experience of the problem in their community [27]. Country health services of LAMIC are generally ill-equipped to meet the needs of older persons. Health care, even at the primary care level, is clinic-based: the older person must attend the clinic, often involving a long journey and waiting time in the clinic, to receive care. Even if they can get to the clinic, the assessment and treatment that they receive is oriented towards acute rather than chronic conditions. The perception is that the former may be treatable, the latter intractable and not within the realm of responsibility of health services [56].

Efforts to increase demand for dementia care through improved awareness must be accompanied by health system and service reform, so that help-seeking is met with a supply of better-prepared, more responsive services. In parallel with its epidemiological surveys, the 10/66 Dementia Research Group has been testing the effectiveness of training community healthcare workers to identify people with dementia [57–59], and to deliver a brief intervention to educate and train carers [20]. Initial findings, from the first two of several randomized controlled trials of the 10/66 Helping Carers to Care intervention, in Goa [60] and in Moscow [61], show highly promising results. The WHO has launched a Mental Health Gap Action Program (mhGAP) to scale up care for mental, neurological, and substance use disorders, and to reduce the treatment gap [62]. Dementia is one of the seven priority areas, along with depression, psychosis, epilepsy, child and adolescent disorders, alcohol use, and suicide. Evidence-based guidelines for treatment and care by non-specialists are being prepared, with the aim of implementing and evaluating them in selected LAMIC. Some of those involved with the mhGAP work on dementia published preliminary proposals for evidence-based packages of care as part of a concurrent *PLÓS Medicine* series [63]. Recommendations are that

1. Routine packages of continuing care should comprise diagnosis coupled with information, regular needs assessments, physical health checks, and carer support, and where necessary carer training, respite care, and assessment and treatment of BPSD.
2. Care can be delivered by trained primary care teams working in a collaborative care framework.
3. Continuing care with practice-based care coordination, and community outreach are essential components of this model.
4. Efficient care delivery in LAMIC involves integrating dementia care with that of other chronic diseases and community-support programs for the elderly and disabled.

Future priorities

Clearly progress has been made. A recent *Lancet Neurology* review [64] chronicles both the growing awareness of the importance of dementia in LAMIC, and the burgeoning evidence base. Having clarified the prevalence and impact of dementia in LAMIC, there is now a need to shift focus to possibilities for prevention, and improvements in delivery of care.

Prevention

The 10/66 Dementia Research Group is currently engaged in a three-year incidence phase follow-up of the baseline sample. The incidence phase will exploit the rich baseline cross-sectional data in the six Latin American countries (Cuba, Dominican Republic, Venezuela, Mexico, Peru, and Argentina) and in China to assess risk factors for incident dementia, stroke, and mortality. Verbal autopsy will be used to identify causes of death. The incidence phase will involve approximately 15 000 older people, and will be completed by mid 2010. We will estimate the annual incidence rate of dementia and its subtypes, by age group, education, and center, and investigate risk factors for incident dementia and Alzheimer's disease, focusing upon cardiovascular risk factors, micronutrient deficiencies and other dietary deficiencies, anemia, and subclinical hypothyroidism. We will also seek to confirm in all sites the predictive validity of the survey dementia diagnoses (DSM-IV and "the 10/66 dementia algorithm') and MCI through three-year follow-up of all dementia and MCI cases, and to carry out a longitudinal study of evolving care arrangements for people with dementia, and carer strain.

Treatment and care

The effectiveness of the 10/66 "Helping Carers to Care" intervention, provisionally demonstrated in Russia and in India, is being further tested in randomized controlled trials in Peru, Mexico, Venezuela, the Dominican Republic, and China; when these are complete the results will be meta-analysed across all seven trials [20]. With support from ADI, the fully manualized intervention package, and two-day training program supported by a training DVD is being made available in English, Latin American (Spanish), Indian (Tamil and Hindi), and Chinese versions. More work will need to be done to support the effective implementation of the mhGAP treatment package. The lack of a suitably brief and cross-culturally validated screening assessment for use in primary care has been highlighted [63]. Physical health assessments and "dementia screens" (to exclude common secondary causes) are routinely advocated in high income countries [65], but there is no evidence for their cost-effectiveness in LAMIC. Cognitive stimulation, and reminiscence therapy seem potentially promising components of a package of care, particularly if carers could be trained to administer simplified versions of these interventions in the home setting [63]. The overall effectiveness and cost-effectiveness of the whole mhGAP dementia package will need to be demonstrated if policy makers are to be persuaded to invest scarce healthcare resources. Most importantly, fundamental health system reform – a partial reorientation towards chronic disease care coupled with appropriate workforce training – is necessary and overdue [66].

References

1. The 10/66 Dementia Research Group. Dementia in Developing Countries. A preliminary consensus statement from the 10/66 Dementia Research Group. *Int J Geriatr Psychiatry* 2000; **15**: 14–20.

2. The 10/66 Dementia Research Group. Methodological issues in population-based research into dementia in developing countries. A position paper from the 10/66 Dementia Research Group. *Int J Geriatr Psychiatry* 2000; **15**: 21–30.

3. Prince M, Acosta D, Chiu H, Scazufca M, Varghese M. Dementia diagnosis in developing countries: a cross-cultural validation study. *Lancet* 2003; **361**(9361): 909–17.

4. Liu S I, Prince M, Chiu MJ, *et al.* Validity and reliability of a Taiwan Chinese version of the community screening instrument for dementia. *Am J Geriatr Psychiatry* 2005; **13**(7): 581–8.

5. Copeland JRM, Dewey ME, Griffith-Jones HM. A computerised psychiatric diagnostic system and case nomenclature for elderly subjects: GMS and AGECAT. *Psychol Med* 1986; **16**: 89–99.

6. Hall KS, Hendrie HH, Brittain HM, *et al.* The development of a dementia screening interview in two distinct languages. *Int J Methods Psychiatr Res* 1993; **3**:1–28.
7. Ganguli M, Chandra V, Gilby JE, *et al.* Cognitive test performance in a community-based nondemented elderly sample in rural India: the Indo-U.S. Cross-National Dementia Epidemiology Study. *Int Psychogeriatr* 1996; **8**(4): 507–24.
8. American Psychiatric Association. *Diagnostic and Statistical Manual of Mental Disorders*, 4th edn. Washington, DC, American Psychiatric Association, 1994.
9. Prince M, Rodriguez JL, Noriega L, *et al.* The 10/66 Dementia Research Group's fully operationalized DSM IV dementia computerized diagnostic algorithm, compared with the 10/66 dementia algorithm and a clinician diagnosis: a population validation study. *BMC Public Health* 2008; **8**: 219.
10. Hendrie HC, Osuntokun BO, Hall KS, *et al.* Prevalence of Alzheimer's disease and dementia in two communities: Nigerian Africans and African Americans. *Am J Psychiatry* 1995; **152**: 1485–92.
11. Chandra V, Ganguli M, Pandav R, *et al.* Prevalence of Alzheimer's disease and other dementias in rural India. The Indo-US study. *Neurology* 1998; **51**: 1000–8.
12. Joteeshwaran AT, Williams JD, Prince MJ. The predictive validity of the 10/66 Dementia diagnosis in Chennai, India – a three year follow-up study of cases identified at baseline. *Alzheimer Dis Assoc Disord.* In press 2009.
13. Ferri CP, Prince M, Brayne C, *et al.* Global prevalence of dementia: a Delphi consensus study. *Lancet* 2005; **366**(9503): 2112–17.
14. World Health Organization. *The Atlas of Heart Disease and Stroke*. Geneva, World Health Organization, 2004.
15. Hendrie HC, Ogunniyi A, Hall KS, *et al.* Incidence of dementia and Alzheimer disease in 2 communities: Yoruba residing in Ibadan, Nigeria, and African Americans residing in Indianapolis, Indiana.[see comment]. *JAMA* 2001; **285**(6): 739–47.
16. Chandra V, Pandav R, Dodge HH, *et al.* Incidence of Alzheimer's disease in a rural community in India: the Indo-US study. *Neurology* 2001; **57**(6): 985–9.
17. Herrera E Jr, Caramelli P, Silveira AS, Nitrini R. Epidemiologic survey of dementia in a community-dwelling Brazilian population. *Alzheimer Dis Assoc Disord* 2002; **16**(2): 103–8.
18. Nitrini R, Caramelli P, Herrera E Jr, *et al.* Incidence of dementia in a community-dwelling Brazilian population. *Alzheimer Dis Assoc Disord* 2004; **18**(4): 241–6.
19. Rosselli D, Ardila A, Pradilla G, *et al.* [The Mini-Mental State Examination as a selected diagnostic test for dementia: a Colombian population study. GENECO]. *Rev Neurol* 2000; **30**(5): 428–32.
20. Prince M, Ferri CP, Acosta D, *et al.* The protocols for the 10/66 Dementia Research Group population-based research program. *BMC Public Health* 2007; **7**(1): 165.
21. Llibre Rodriguez JJ, Ferri CP, Acosta D, *et al.* Prevalence of dementia in Latin America, India and China: a population-based cross-sectional survey. *Lancet* 2008; **372**(9637): 464–74.
22. Scazufca M, Menezes PR, Vallada HP, *et al.* High prevalence of dementia among older adults from poor socioeconomic backgrounds in Sao Paulo, Brazil. *Int Psychogeriatr* 2008; **20**(2): 394–405.

23. Llibre RJ, Valhuerdi A, Sanchez II, *et al.* The prevalence, correlates and impact of dementia in Cuba. A 10/66 group population-based survey. *Neuroepidemiology* 2008; **31**(4): 243–51.

24. Acosta D, Rottbeck R, Rodriguez G, Ferri CP, Prince MJ. The epidemiology of dependency among urban-dwelling older people in the Dominican Republic; a cross-sectional survey. *BMC Public Health* 2008; **8**(1): 285.

25. Jacob KS, Kumar PS, Gayathri K, Abraham S, Prince MJ. The diagnosis of dementia in the community. *Int Psychogeriatr* 2007; **19**(4): 669–78.

26. Shaji KS, Smitha K, Praveen Lal K, Prince M. Caregivers of people with Alzheimer's disease: a qualitative study from the Indian 10/66 Dementia Research Network. *Int J Geriatr Psychiatry* 2002; **18**: 1–6.

27. Patel V, Prince M. Ageing and mental health in a developing country: who cares? Qualitative studies from Goa, India. *Psychol Med* 2001; **31**(1): 29–38.

28. Lobo A, Saz P, Marcos G, *et al.* Prevalence of dementia in a southern European population in two different time periods: the ZARADEMP Project. *Acta Psychiatr Scand* 2007; **116**(4): 299–307.

29. Fernandez M, Castro-Flores J, Perez-de las HS, *et al.* [Prevalence of dementia in the elderly aged above 65 in a district in the Basque Country.] *Rev Neurol* 2008; **46**(2): 89–96.

30. Francesconi P, Roti L, Casotto V, *et al.* [Prevalence of dementia in Tuscany: results from four population-based epidemiological studies.] *Epidemiol Prev* 2006; **30**(4–5): 237–44.

31. Plassman BL, Langa KM, Fisher GG, *et al.* Prevalence of dementia in the United States: the aging, demographics, and memory study. *Neuroepidemiology* 2007; **29**(1–2): 125–32.

32. Bottino CM, Azevedo D Jr, Tatsch M, *et al.* Estimate of dementia prevalence in a community sample from Sao Paulo, Brazil. *Dement Geriatr Cogn Disord* 2008; **26**(4): 291–9.

33. Custodio N. Prevalencia de demencia en una comunidad urbana de Lima: Un estudio puerta a puerta. (Abstract). Santo Domingo, Republica Dominicana, XII Congreso Panamericano de Neurologia, 2007.

34. Llibre JJ, Fernández Y, Marcheco B, Contreras N, López AM, Ote M. Prevalence of dementia and Alzheimer's disease in a Havana municipality: A community-based study among elderly residents. *MEDICC Rev* 2009; **11**(2): 29–35.

35. Molero AE, Pino-Ramirez G, Maestre GE. High prevalence of dementia in a Caribbean population. *Neuroepidemiology* 2007; **29**(1–2): 107–12.

36. Zhang ZX, Zahner GE, Roman GC, *et al.* Socio-demographic variation of dementia subtypes in china: Methodology and results of a prevalence study in Beijing, Chengdu, Shanghai, and Xian. *Neuroepidemiology* 2006; **27**(4): 177–87.

37. Jhoo JH, Kim KW, Huh Y, *et al.* Prevalence of dementia and its subtypes in an elderly urban korean population: results from the Korean Longitudinal Study on Health And Aging (KLoSHA). *Dement Geriatr Cogn Disord* 2008; **26**(3): 270–6.

38. Shaji S, Bose S, Verghese A. Prevalence of dementia in an urban population in Kerala, India. *Br J Psychiatry* 2005; **186**: 136–40.

39. Wangtongkum S, Sucharitkul P, Silprasert N, Inthrachak R. Prevalence of dementia among population age over 45 years in Chiang Mai, Thailand. *J Med Assoc Thai* 2008; **91**(11): 1685–90.

40. Smith K, Flicker L, Lautenschlager NT, *et al.* High prevalence of dementia and cognitive

impairment in Indigenous Australians. *Neurology* 2008; **71**(19): 1470–3.

41. Galasko D, Salmon D, Gamst A, *et al.* Prevalence of dementia in Chamorros on Guam: relationship to age, gender, education, and APOE. *Neurology* 2007; **68**(21): 1772–81.
42. Bdzan LB, Turczynski J, Szabert K. [Prevalence of dementia in a rural population.] *Psychiatr Pol* 2007; **41**(2): 181–8.
43. Gurvit H, Emre M, Tinaz S, *et al.* The prevalence of dementia in an urban Turkish population. *Am J Alzheimers Dis Other Demen* 2008; **23**(1): 67–76.
44. Alzheimer's Disease International. *World Alzheimer Report 2009.* London, Alzheimer's Disease International, 2009.
45. Prince M. Commentary: Two-phase surveys. A death is announced; no flowers please. *Int J Epidemiol* 2003; **32**(6): 1078–80.
46. Choo WY, Low WY, Karina R, *et al.* Social support and burden among caregivers of patients with dementia in Malaysia. *Asia Pac J Public Health* 2003; **15**(1): 23–9.
47. Dias A, Samuel R, Patel V, *et al.* The impact associated with caring for a person with dementia: a report from the 10/66 Dementia Research Group's Indian network. *Int J Geriatr Psychiatry* 2004; **19**(2): 182–4.
48. 10/66 Dementia Research Group. Care arrangements for people with dementia in developing countries. *Int J Geriatr Psychiatry* 2004; **19**(2): 170–7.
49. Tout K. *Ageing in Developing Countries.* Oxford, Oxford University Press, 1989.
50. Prince M, Acosta D, Albanese E, *et al.* Ageing and dementia in low and middle income countries-Using research to engage with public and policy makers. *Int Rev Psychiatry* 2008; **20**(4): 332–43.
51. Prince MJ. The 10/66 dementia research group – 10 years on. *Indian J Psychiatry* 2009; **51**: S8–15.
52. Ferri CP, Ames D, Prince M. Behavioral and psychological symptoms of dementia in developing countries. *Int Psychogeriatr* 2004; **16**(4): 441–59.
53. Sousa RM, Ferri CP, Acosta D, *et al.* Contribution of chronic diseases to disability in elderly people in countries with low and middle incomes: a 10/66 Dementia Research Group population-based survey. *Lancet* 2009; **374** (9704): 1821–30.
54. Wimo A, Winblad B, Jonsson L. An estimate of the total worldwide societal costs of dementia in 2005. *Alzheimers Dement* 2007; **3**(2): 81–91.
55. Cohen L. Toward an anthropology of senility: anger, weakness, and Alzheimer's in Banaras, India. *Med Anthropol Q* 1995; **9**(3): 314–34.
56. Prince M, Livingston G, Katona C. Mental health care for the elderly in low-income countries: a health systems approach. *World Psychiatry* 2007; **6**(1): 5–13.
57. Shaji KS, Arun Kishore NR, Lal KP, Prince M. Revealing a hidden problem. An evaluation of a community dementia case-finding program from the Indian 10/66 dementia research network. *Int J Geriatr Psychiatry* 2002; **17**(3): 222–5.
58. Ramos-Cerqueira AT, Torres AR, Crepaldi AL, *et al.* Identification of dementia cases in the community: a Brazilian experience. *J Am Geriatr Soc* 2005; **53**(10): 1738–42.
59. Jacob KS, Senthil KP, Gayathri K, Abraham S, Prince MJ. Can health workers diagnose dementia in the community? *Acta Psychiatr Scand* 2007; **116**(2): 125–8.
60. Dias A, Dewey ME, D'Souza J, *et al.* The effectiveness of a home care program for

supporting caregivers of persons with dementia in developing countries: a randomized controlled trial from Goa, India. *PLoS ONE* 2008; **3**(6): e2333.

61. Gavrilova SI, Ferri CP, Mikhaylova N, *et al.* Helping carers to care–the 10/66 dementia research group's randomized control trial of a caregiver intervention in Russia. *Int J Geriatr Psychiatry* 2009; **24**(4): 347–54.
62. World Health Organization. mhGAP: Mental Health Gap Action Programme: scaling up care for mental, neurological and substance use disorders. Geneva, World Health Organization, 2008.
63. Prince MJ, Acosta D, Castro-Costa E, Jackson J, Shaji KS. Packages of care for dementia in low- and middle-income countries. *PLoS Med* 2009; **6**(11): e1000176.
64. Kalaria RN, Maestre GE, Arizaga R, *et al.* Alzheimer's disease and vascular dementia in developing countries: prevalence, management, and risk factors. *Lancet Neurol* 2008; **7**(9): 812–26.
65. National Collaborating Centre for Mental Health. Dementia: A NICE-SCIE Guideline on supporting people with dementia and their carers in health and social care. National Clinical Practice Guideline Number 42. Leicester, The British Psychological Society and The Royal College of Psychiatrists, 2007.
66. Beaglehole R, Ebrahim S, Reddy S, Voute J, Leeder S. Prevention of chronic diseases: a call to action. *Lancet* 2007; **370**(9605): 2152–7.

Further reading

Amella E, & NICHE Faculty. Assessment and management of eating and feeding difficulties for older people: a NICHE protocol. *Geriatr Nurs* 1998; **19**(5): 269–74.

Assal F, Cummings JL. Neuropsychiatric symptoms in the dementias. *Curr Opin Neurol* 2002; **15**: 445–50.

Ballard CG, Gauthier S, Cummings JL, *et al.* Management of agitation and aggression associated with Alzheimer disease. *Nat Rev Neurol* 2009; **5**: 245–55.

Biessels GJ, Koffeman A, Scheltens P. Diabetes and cognitive impairment: clinical diagnosis and brain imaging in patients attending a memory clinic. *J Neurol* 2006; **253**: 477–82.

Bruen PD, McGeown WJ, Shanks MF, Venneri A. Neuroanatomical correlates of neuropsychiatric symptoms in Alzheimer's disease. *Brain* 2008; **131**: 2455–63.

Caris-Verhallen W, Kerkstra A, Bensing J. Non-verbal behaviour in nurse-elderly patient communication. *J Adv Nurs* 1999; **29**(4): 808–18.

Cohen-Mansfield J, Werner, Marx MS. Screaming in nursing home residents. *J Am Geriatr Soc* 1990; **38**: 785–92.

Cummings JL, Schneider E, Tariot PN, Graham SM, for the Memantine MEM-MD-02 Study Group. Behavioral effects of memantine in Alzheimer disease patients receiving donepezil treatment. *Neurology* 2006; **67**: 57–63.

Franceschi M, Anchisi D, Pelati O, *et al.* Glucose metabolism and serotonin receptors in the frontotemporal lobe degeneration. *Ann Neurol* 2005; **57**: 216–25.

Gauthier S, Feldman H, Hecker J, *et al.* Efficacy of donepezil on behavioural symptoms in patients with moderate to severe Alzheimer's disease. *Int Psychogeriatr* 2002; **14**: 389–404.

Glinn NJ. The music therapy assessment tool in Alzheimer's patients. *J Gerontol Nurs* 1992; **18**: 3–9.

Hendryx-Bedalov PM. Alzheimer's dementia: coping with communication decline. *J Gerontol Nurs* 2000; **26**(8): 20–4.

Herbert C. Assessing nutrition in elderly patients. *Nurs Stand* 1996; **10**(17): 35–7.

Hirono N, Mega MS, Dinov ID, Mishkin F, Cummings JL. Left frontotemporal hypoperfusion is associated with aggression in patients with dementia. *Arch Neurology* 2000; **57**: 861–6.

Hirono N, Mori E, Ishii K, *et al.* Frontal lobe hypometabolism and depression in Alzheimer's disease. *Neurology* 1998; **50**: 380–3.

Jacelon, C. Preventing cascade iatrogenesis in hospitalized elders: an important role for nurses. *J Gerontol Nurs* 1999; **25**(1): 27–33.

Knopnan DS, Sawyer-DeMaris S. Practical approaches to managing behavioral problems in dementia patients. *Geriatrics* 1990; **45**: 25–37.

Kowanko, I. The role of the nurse in food service: a literature review and recommendations. *Int J Nurs Pract* 1997; **3**(2): 73–8.

Kowanko I, Simon S, Wood J. Nutritional care of the patient: nurses' knowledge and attitudes in an acute care setting. *J Clin Nurs* 1999; **8**: 217–24.

Liu W, Miller BL, Krammer JH, *et al.* Behavioral disorders in the frontal and temporal variants of frontotemporal dementia. *Neurology* 2004; **62**: 742–8.

Malone KM, Mann JJ. Neuroanatomic correlates of psychopathologic components of major depressive disorder. *Arch Gen Psychiatry* 2005; **62**: 397–408.

Mann JJ. The medical management of depression. *N Engl J Med* 2005; **353**(17): 1819–34

Marcus E, Berry E. Refusal to eat in the elderly. *Nutr Rev* 1998; **56**(6): 163–71.

McMurray AM, Chen AK, Shapira IS, *et al.* Variation in regional SPECT hypoperfusion and clinical features in frontotemporal dementia. *Neurology* 2006; **66**: 517–22.

Meeks TW, Ropacki SA, Jeste DV. The neurobiology of neuropsychiatric syndromes in dementia. *Curr Opin Psychiatry* 2006; **19**: 581–6.

Mendez MF, McMurtray A, Chen AK, *et al.* Functional neuroimaging and presenting psychiatric features in frontotemporal dementia. *J Neurol Neurosurg Psychiatry* 2006; **77**: 4–7.

Phillips VL, Diwan S. The incremental effect of dementia-related problem behaviors on the time to nursing home placement in poor, frail, demented older people. *J Am Geriatr Soc* 2003; **51**: 188–93.

Prince M, Acosta D, Chiu H. Dementia Diagnosis in developing countries. A cross-cultural validation study. *Lancet* 2003; **361**(9361): 909–17.

Rajkumar S, Hoolahan B. Remoteness and issues in mental health care: experience from rural Australia. *Epidemiol Psichiatr Soc* 2004; **13**(2): 78–82.

Sammut A. Dementia and challenging behaviours: a person centred approach to care. *National ACA/AAG Conference Paper*, Sydney, September 8, 1999 (paper supplied by author).

Schneider LS, Dagerman KS, Insel P. Risk of death with atypical antipsychotic drug treatment for dementia. Meta-analysis of randomized placebo-controlled trials. *JAMA* 2005; **294**: 1934–43.

Sultzer D, Brown CV, Mandelkern MA, *et al.* Delusional thoughts and regional frontal/temporal cortex metabolism in Alzheimer's disease. *Am J Psychiatry* 2003; **160**: 341–9.

Sweet RA, Nimgaonkar VL, Devlin B, Jeste D. Psychiatric symptoms in Alzheimer's disease: evidence for a distinct phenotype. *Mol Psychiatry* 2003; **8**: 383–92.

Strumpf, N. Improving care for the frail elderly. *J Gerontol Nurs* 2000; **26**(7): 37–43.

Trinh NH, Hoblyn J, Mahanty S, Yaffe K. Efficacy of cholinesterase inhibitors in the treatment of neuropsychiatric symptoms and functional impairment in Alzheimer's disease. *JAMA* 2003; **289**: 210–16.

Tsang SW, Vinters HV, Cummings JL, *et al.* Alteration in NMDA receptor subunit densities and ligand binding to glycine recognition sites are associated with chronic anxiety in Alzheimer's disease. *Neurobiol Aging* 2008; **29**: 1524–32.

Zaudig M. A new systematic method of measurement and diagnosis of mild cognitive impairment and dementia according to ICD-10 and DSM-III R criteria. *Int Psychogeriatr* 1992; **4**: 203–19.

Index

Page numbers in italics indicate items in tables